The Sexual Brain

The Sexual Brain

Simon LeVay

A Bradford Book
The MIT Press
Cambridge, Massachusetts
London, England

First MIT Press paperback edition, 1994

This book was set in Sabon by .eps Electronic Publishing Services and was printed and bound in the United States of America.

Library of Congress Cataloging-in-Publication Data

LeVay, Simon.
  The sexual brain / Simon LeVay.
    p. cm.
  "A Bradford book."
  Includes bibliographical references and index.
  ISBN 0-262-12178-6 (HB), 0-262-62093-6 (PB)
    1. Neuropsychology. 2. Brain—Sex differences. 3. Sex.
I. Title.
QP360.L4926 1993   92-44691
155.3′3—dc20   CIP

In memory of Richard George Hersey

Contents

Acknowledgments

First, I am grateful to Chuck Stevens for suggesting that I write this book.

Second, I owe a major debt to six individuals who read earlier versions of the manuscript and provided many valuable suggestions for improvement. They are Michael Bailey (Northwestern University), Marc Breedlove (University of California, Berkeley), Dean Hamer (National Cancer Institute), Darcy Kelly (Columbia University), Jeremy Nathans (Johns Hopkins University), and Fiona Stevens of The MIT Press.

Finally, I thank the Salk Institute for paying more than lip service to the notion of academic freedom.

Introduction

O, then I see Queen Mab hath been with you.
She is the fairies' midwife, and she comes
In shape no bigger than an agate stone
On the forefinger of an alderman,
Drawn with a team of little atomies
Athwart men's noses as they lie asleep;
Her wagon spokes made of long spinners' legs,
The cover, of the wings of grasshoppers;
Her traces, of the smallest spider's web;
Her collars, of the moonshine's wat'ry beams;
Her whip, of cricket's bone; the lash, of film;
Her wagoner, a small grey-coated gnat,
Not half so big as a round little worm
Pricked from the lazy finger of a maid;
Her chariot is an empty hazelnut,
Made by the joiner squirrel or old grub,
Time out o' mind the fairies' coachmakers.
And in this state she gallops night by night
Through lovers' brains, and then they dream of love . . .
—William Shakespeare, *Romeo and Juliet,* I.iv

In the passage quoted above, Mercutio offers Romeo an explanation for his amorous feelings that is as inaccurate as it is romantic. Yet in one respect Mercutio was closer to the truth than many of his contemporaries: he located these feelings, not in the heart, liver, or bowels, but in the brain.

The aim of this book is to focus more precisely on the brain mechanisms that are responsible for sexual behavior and feelings. Because there are such striking individual differences in sexuality—most obviously between men and women, but also among individuals of the same sex—one of the book's major concerns is to look for the biological basis for this diversity.

Until recently, the study of human sexuality has been mainly the province of *psychology,* the academic discipline devoted to the study of the mind. Psychology itself should logically be thought of as a division of *biology,* the scientific study of life as a whole. Yet for too long psychology existed as a self-contained discipline, answerable to no other laws than its own. Its tools were primarily talk and the observation of behavior. When scientists carrying microscopes and electrodes turned their attention to the brain, it did not occur to them to call themselves psychologists, even though they knew that they were studying the mechanisms of mental life. They called themselves *neurobiologists* instead.

So different have been these two approaches to the mind, that the belief has arisen that they offer mutually exclusive explanations for mental processes. People will ask of some trait—homosexuality, for example—"Is it psychological or is it biological?" By that they generally mean "Is it some nebulous state of mind resulting from upbringing and social interactions, or is it a matter of genes and brain chemistry?" But this is a false distinction, since even the most nebulous and socially determined states of mind are a matter of genes and brain chemistry too.

I myself have fallen into this error. In 1991 I published a study in which I described a difference in brain structure between homosexual and heterosexual men. As the last sentence of the summary of the paper, I wrote: "This finding . . . suggests that sexual orientation has a biological substrate." By that, I was implying that there are some aspects of mental life that do *not* have a biological substrate—an absurd idea, and one that is implicitly rejected even in Mercutio's philosophy.

The real difference between psychology and neurobiology is this: traditionally, psychologists attempted to reduce complex mental processes to processes that were simpler but still by their nature *mental.* Although they may never have said as much, their Holy Grail was the "elementary particle" of mentation. Neurobiologists, on the other hand, have tried to explain mental processes in terms of simpler, *nonmental* processes, like those studied by physicists and chemists. This difference of approach led naturally to conflict. As psychologists saw it, neurobiologists were ignoring—perhaps even challenging the existence of—those very aspects of mental life, such as consciousness, that make it such an interesting phenomenon. To neurobiologists, on the other hand, it seemed that psychologists had an undue reverence for the mind as something mysteriously elevated above the humdrum world of causes and effects.

To some extent this conflict has been resolved over the past decade. Terms like "biological psychology" or "psychobiology" reflect a new desire to combine the two disciplines. In this book, I have not totally ignored psychological studies of sex, even though I am a neurobiologist by training and sympathy. But the emphasis is on understanding sex in terms of the cellular processes that generate it.

Although my 1991 study of the hypothalamus of gay and straight men generated a great deal of media attention and public interest, it is actually my only research publication on the subject of sex, to date at least, and it took up a mere three pages in the journal *Science*. My research previously was directed at another mental function, vision. Over the years, I have studied the structure, function, and development of the visual areas of the cerebral cortex. I have been particularly interested in the question of how the inputs from the two eyes are integrated by the brain into a single view of the world. On the face of it, then, I am not especially qualified to write a book on sex.

At another level, though, circumstances have conspired to make writing this book an especially appropriate task for me. For one thing, as a gay man I have always had a personal interest in sexuality in general, and in sexual orientation in particular. As a teenager and young adult I accepted the Freudian line, according to which a young child's relations with his or her parents play a decisive role. For one thing, it was the dominant idea in the 1960s. For another, it seemed to be borne out in my own family experience: I remembered my mother as having been very close and possessive, and my father as distant, even hostile. This is exactly the kind of family environment which, according Freud, makes it difficult for young boys to follow the "normal" path to heterosexuality. And when I came to read Freud I was swept away by his eloquence and the sheer audacity of his theories.

Later, though, I began to have serious doubts. First, as I got to know large numbers of gay men and lesbian women, it became harder and harder to see them, or myself, as the products of defective parenting; we just seemed too normal. Second, as I became trained in the methods of science I became more and more skeptical that there was anything scientific about Freud's ideas, even though he repeatedly asserted that they were so. And finally, discoveries were being made in the area of sexual biology that were pointing in all kinds of new and exciting directions; Freudianism, on the other hand, seemed to have become a fossilized, immovable dogma.

When, as a postdoctoral fellow and junior faculty member, I worked in the laboratory of David Hubel and Torsten Wiesel at Harvard Medical School, I was particularly influenced by their research on the development of the visual system. They found that the visual system of a newly born monkey is remarkably similar to that of an adult; to a large extent, the system assembles itself prenatally, before the monkey has seen anything. Far from being a blank slate, the newborn monkey's mind is prejudiced to see the world in the way that monkeys do see the world, because of the nature of the wiring already present in its brain. They went on to show that a mutation in just one gene could radically alter the functional organization of the visual cortex. On the basis of these findings, and those of many other researchers, it seemed reasonable to ask whether inborn differences in brain organization, at least partly under genetic control, might not be the basis of the diversity of many mental functions in humans, including those related to sex.

Because I only became a sex researcher so recently, I have maintained a certain amateurish or journalistic attitude to the field. This may have some negative consequences; for example, there may be more sheer errors of fact than are usual in a book of this type, and if so, I apologize for them. But my newness to the field has allowed me, I think, to view it with a certain innocent enthusiasm that is difficult to preserve over the years: in any field of study one eventually gets weighed down, paralyzed even, by the sheer mass of conflicting findings and theories. I have not yet reached that point.

Although my own special interest has to do with the issue of sexual orientation, this book is not focused primarily on that topic. Rather it deals broadly with sexuality from a biological point of view. It tackles the subject in a sequence of stages, beginning with broad concepts and homing in on specific issues later.

In the first chapter I bring up the question of nature-versus-nurture—that is, the relative roles of hereditary and environmental factors in sexuality. The second chapter is a discussion of the evolutionary forces that have made us into sexual creatures and molded our sexual behavior. In the third chapter, I describe how our bodies develop as male or female. Chapter 4 finally introduces the brain; this chapter is an essay in which I try to illustrate the main features of brain organization, as we presently understand it. I present the main lines of evidence for regional specialization of function in the brain. The next chapter focuses on the hypothalamus, the brain region most intimately involved in the production of sexual behavior and feelings. Chapter 6 is devoted to the actual mechanics of sex and the neural mechanisms that control them. The following two chapters discuss two sex-differentiated traits—courtship and maternal behavior—whose basis in brain function has been studied in a variety of animals. Then in chapter 9 I present the evidence that sexual behaviors typical of males and females depend on the function of distinct, specialized regions within the hypothalamus. Chapter 10 is devoted to the development of these brain regions in males and females. I discuss the evidence that the brain, like the body, is intrinsically female: male brain traits require the presence of specific hormonal signals at certain times during development. In chapter 11 I briefly discuss some of the differences between men and women that fall outside the sphere of sex itself, and how these differences may arise. Chapter 12, by far the longest in the book, deals with sexual orientation. In this chapter I attempt to bring together many of the themes covered earlier to present as balanced a picture as possible of the biological mechanisms that may contribute to making a person gay, straight, or bisexual. In chapter 13 I touch on the thorny issue of gender identity: What is it that leads us to believe we are male or female? Finally, in the Epilogue I briefly sum up the book and revisit the nature-versus-nurture debate.

I have tried to write this book in such a way as to make it accessible to any interested reader. As much as I have been able, I have explained all technical terms where they first appear, and have assumed no more knowledge on the reader's part than I have already presented. There may be points where the reader feels that the going has become excessively technical, or where the relevance to the main theme may not yet be evident. I hope that the coherence of the diverse themes will become evident as the reader progresses. I have also written summary paragraphs for many of the chapters, either at the end of the chapter or at the beginning of the following chapter. If a particular chapter does not interest you, or seems too technical, I suggest you read the summary and go on to the next topic. I also recommend the use of the Glossary if the meaning of a term is unclear.

1

Thou, Nature, Art My Goddess

Genes, Environment, and Sex

There are two broad classes of ideas—two prejudices, if you like—that characterize people's attitude toward sexuality and its development. One is that we are all born with very similar brains. According to this prejudice, our individual sexual lives, both our inner lives of desires, inhibitions, and fulfillment, and our external life of sexual and reproductive activity, are molded by outside inputs to the brain: by our realization, from looking at our bodies as young children, of which sex we are, and by the influence of parents, family, teachers, sexual partners, and society in general. The opposite prejudice is that each person's brain is preprogrammed to function in a characteristic sexual mode—male or female, gay or straight, promiscuous or celibate—and that these characteristics will emerge whatever the environment.

The conflict between these two points of view is an example of the age-old *nature-versus-nurture* controversy that has raged since before biology became a science. The extreme positions are of course untenable: genes cannot operate in a vacuum, nor can the environment mold a sentient, behaving being out of nothingness. But we are not concerned with extremes; we are concerned with the inborn differences between individuals that may reasonably exist, and the range of environments to which these individuals may reasonably be exposed. Within this more limited context the nature/nurture debate is still unresolved for most aspects of human behavior, and it provides the appropriate framework to think about sex.

In my view, the scientific evidence presently available points to a strong influence of nature, and only a modest influence of nurture. This view conflicts with the beliefs of most lay people, as well as many professionals, who generally place stress on external factors, such as the environment or family relations, as the determinants of a person's sexuality as well as other aspects of character and behavior.

The widespread tendency to exaggerate the importance of environment in development has several causes. First, children develop slowly: they do everything clumsily at first, and then better. During this period of improving performance, their parents are lovingly "teaching" them—to walk, for example, by holding them up with two hands, then one hand, a finger, letting them take one step alone, two, and so on. It is impossible for most parents to believe that if they had never bothered themselves with their child's locomotion, he or she would have made the transition from crawling to walking unaided. Yet this is what the child probably would have done.

What about a more cultural trait, such as language? Of course, a child would never come to speak English if he or she did not hear English spoken. To that extent, language acquisition clearly involves imitation—an interaction with the environment. Nevertheless, it is becoming widely accepted that children are born in possession of extensive information about the general structure of human language, and cannot learn any of the many possible languages that violate this structure. Equipped with this information, a child can readily pick up the the verbal patterns of any particular human language.

The other reason for overestimating the role of the environment is simply wishful thinking. Parents naturally like to take the credit for their children's achievements and fine character, and if their achievements are few or their character flawed, other environmental influences such as school or TV can always take the blame. Most people think nurture is fairer than nature: allowing inborn factors a leading role seems to load the dice in the game of life. Yet nothing could be as unfair as the differences in *nurture* that exist even between siblings in the same family, let alone between rich and poor, black and white, and so on. Life *is* unfair, from the moment that chance deals you your genes to the moment some random disease or accident kills you.

In humans, as in many other species, there are two sexes, male and female. But how does one judge the sex of a particular individual? When the midwife dangles a newborn infant and declares "It's a girl!" or "It's a boy!," that judgement is based on external anatomy: if the baby has a penis and scrotum then it's a boy, if a clitoris, labial folds, and vagina then it's a girl. These differences in the external genitalia remain the commonly accepted criteria for defining sex, not only among lay people, but also among sexologists and scientists generally. No matter what your chromosomes, no matter what your internal organs, no matter whether you have a beard or breasts, no matter what you call yourself, how you dress or who you lust after—if you have a penis you are a man, if you have a vagina you are a woman.

Of course, these other attributes are generally linked to a person's sex. A man usually (but not always) has one X and one Y sex chromosome in his body cells, while a woman usually has two X chromosomes. This attribute may be called chromosomal sex. A woman generally has ovaries, uterus, and oviducts, while a man generally has testes, seminal vesicles, prostate gland, and the tubing to go with them. These organs define what might be called an internal sex. After puberty, most men have hairier bodies, deeper voices, and smaller breasts than women (secondary sexual characteristics). Most, but not all, men are sexually attracted to women, and vice versa (sexual orientation). Most men have a deep inner conviction that they are male, and most women that they are female (gender identity). Yet even here there are exceptions: individuals who, in spite of every evidence of their anatomy, in spite of every teaching and pressure of their family and society, and without any sign of mental illness (unless this itself be considered one), are utterly and unshakeably convinced that they belong to the other sex. This phenomenon of transsexuality, although rare, is striking evidence that there is an inner representation of one's sex that can exist independently of any obvious or immediate connection with the world outside the mind.

So the word *sex,* without any qualifier, means sex as defined by the appearance of the external genitalia. Because these other attributes, such as chromosomal patterns or the direction of sexual attraction, are commonly linked to sex, one often talks of a woman (or female animal) with XY sex chromosomes as being "chromosomally male," of a male that has sex with other males as showing "female-typical" sexual behavior, and so on. But these usages are largely a matter of convenience: chromosomes and behaviors themselves have no sex.

Beyond sexual behavior (by which I mean sexual intercourse of any kind, along with behavior related to it such as courtship), there are many other behaviors and cognitive traits that typically show differences be-

tween the sexes. These *sex-differentiated* functions include parental behavior, aggressiveness, visuospatial skills, and so on. Although these
traits have no very direct connection with sex in the narrow sense, the
very fact that they differ between males and females suggests that there
is a biological connection somewhere. I will therefore treat any sex-differentiated trait or behavior as appropriate material for this book.

2

Time's Millioned Accidents
The Evolution of Sex and Sexual Behavior

Ask someone at random what sex is for, and he or she will probably reply: "To keep the human race alive." It is certainly true that if all sexual behavior ceased tomorrow, we would go extinct in short order. This might be the best thing that could happen from the point of view of the general welfare of the planet, but it is not likely to happen, because our genes do not have the general welfare of the planet at heart. Instead they simply propagate themselves under the influence of natural selection, and sex is the way they do it.

But why do they use sex as a means of propagation? Herein lies one of the deepest mysteries of biology. Although sexual reproduction is very common in nature, it is not universal. Some species reproduce *asexually*: that is, a single organism gives rise to progeny without any genetic contribution from another organism. This is true not only of many single-celled species, but also of some higher plants and animals. Dandelions, for example, and certain species of lizards, have completely renounced sex, yet they keep on happily reproducing without suffering any obvious ill-effects of their decision. Many other species can reproduce either sexually or asexually. Given that sex is a fairly cumbersome business, what is the point of it?

One answer to this question can be given at a very general level. Sexual reproduction mixes genes. An asexually produced individual has the same combination of genes as its parent (except for whatever mutations have occurred in the parent's germ line). A sexually produced individual has a different combination of genes from either of its parents (and different from any of its siblings). This variation is the raw material of evolution: it is the means by which advantageous traits, generated at random in unrelated individuals, can be gathered together to create individuals better adapted to their environment.

This argument in favor of sexual reproduction is an argument at the level of the species. Sex may indeed be good for the long-term prospects of the species, but genes do not care about these long-term prospects any more than they care about the general welfare of the planet. Genes demand instant gratification. So what does sex do for the genes that promote sex? To put it more exactly, why has the set of genes that promotes sexual reproduction fared better, in most species, than the alternative set of genes that could have promoted asexual reproduction?

Paradoxically (and herein lies the mystery of sex) there is good reason to believe that the sexual genes should fare *worse* than the asexual genes. To see this, let us imagine a species, like our own, where all individuals are reproducing sexually. One fine day a single female undergoes a mutation such that the entire set of genes for sexual reproduction is replaced by a set of genes for asexual reproduction. (Of course it couldn't happen that neatly, but this is just a thought experiment.) The female then gives birth to offspring who, being just like her, also reproduce asexually. In a population whose overall numbers are stable, each female on average produces two offspring that survive long enough to reproduce. Therefore, other things being equal, the clone of individuals derived from this female, all of whom carry the genes for asexual reproduction, will double its size in each subsequent generation, and eventually the individuals who carry genes for sexual reproduction will be wiped off the face of the earth. No matter that this would hurt the long-term interests of the species: in the short term nothing could stop the runaway expansion of the asexual population and their genes.

Evidently the key phrase here is "other things being equal." They must not be equal, since in general sexual reproduction persists (a few asexual species, such as the lizards mentioned above, presumably did arise from sexual species by a runaway mechanism of this type). There must be some benefit conferred by sexual reproduction that generally ensures the survival of "sexual genes." And we can specify that this benefit must be large enough to double the reproductive success of individuals carrying these genes, compared with individuals carrying the "asexual genes." Only with this much benefit will the sexual genes be able to survive in the face of the asexual genes' ability to expand clonally, that is to double their representation in every generation.

There are two classes of hypotheses for the nature of this benefit. One class looks for the benefit in the interaction of organisms with their environment. These hypotheses start from the fact that sexually generated offspring differ among themselves, and also differ from their parents. Such differences might enhance the average ability of each individual offspring to survive in a variable environment, either because the environment tends to change in unpredictable ways (either in space or time) or because individuals that differ from each other will compete less strongly for limited resources. The latter explanation might be termed the Jack Sprat hypothesis ("Jack Sprat would eat no fat, his wife would eat no lean . . .": their children would likely show a range of fat/lean preferences and hence would fight less over their meals.) Another possibility is that individual animals or plants benefit if their siblings differ in their susceptibility to pathogens or predators. For example, if a particular plant is susceptible to infection by a certain strain of virus, its chances of survival might be reduced if its neighbors (which are likely to be its siblings) share the same susceptibility: they become potential sources of infection.

These environmental hypotheses have a certain plausibility, and in fact there is some experimental evidence to support them. For example, Steven Kelley and his colleagues at Duke University generated sexual and asexual offspring from the same individual plant, and planted them around their parent in a manner simulating the natural dispersion of the plant's offspring. Later he counted the flowers produced by each plant, and found that the sexually generated offspring did significantly better than the asexual offspring. This suggested that some environmental mechanism of the kind just described might be operating. Nevertheless, experiments of this type have not always yielded an appreciable advantage to the sexual progeny, and it is difficult to see why the advantage should be so large and widespread as to make sex the predominant mode of reproduction among higher organisms. If an ecological niche remains constant and unchanged, the organisms that inhabit that niche may also remain relatively unchanged, even for tens or hundreds of millions of years, but the apparent lack of environmental challenge in such a situation doesn't usually cause these species to abandon sex.

The second class of hypotheses views sex as a mechanism to get rid of harmful mutations. When a population reproduces asexually, the number of harmful mutations can never be reduced below the lowest number carried by any individual in the current population. Furthermore, if the population is finite in size, every time another harmful mutation appears in the line with the fewest mutations, that minimum goes up by one and is stuck at this new, higher level. This ratchet-like mechanism was first analyzed by H. J. Muller in the 1960s. Sexually reproducing species, in contrast, can release the ratchet: the random recombination of genes from two parents will generate some offspring who carry fewer harmful mutations than either of their parents.

Clearly then, sexual reproduction can yield some highly advantaged offspring (as well as some highly disadvantaged offspring) compared with those produced asexually, but the important question is: does this translate into a net benefit for the female that chooses the sexual road? To put the question more correctly, does it translate into a net increased survival of the genes that caused her to reproduce sexually, as compared with the survival of the alternative genes that would have caused her to reproduce asexually?

Answering this question is basically a mathematical exercise, but the math has to be applied to some real numbers. Among the numbers we need to know is the average number of new harmful mutations appearing in the germ line of each individual in each generation (more precisely, the average number of harmful mutations an individual inherits from his or her parents that the parents did not inherit from their parents). Traditionally, geneticists have counted mutations by looking for gross abnormalities like fish with three eyes. These mutations are rare (far less than one per lifetime), and therefore they do not provide a sufficient benefit for sexual reproduction to offset the twofold cost mentioned above. But as biologists have developed ever-more-efficient techniques for comparing proteins, sequencing DNA, and so on, it has become apparent that the true mutation rate is much higher, perhaps as much as a hundred or more per individual lifetime. A sizeable fraction of these mutations are likely to be harmful, although the average amount of harm caused by each single mutation may be very slight. With these kinds of numbers, mechanisms to eliminate mutations become much more important.

Besides the actual mutation rate, we also need to know (and this turns out to be crucial) how increasing the number of mutations influences the individual's success at producing offspring (its "fitness"). Is the relationship simply additive—that is, are two mutations exactly twice as bad as one? Or is there "cooperation" between mutations such that two mutations are more than twice as harmful as one? An extreme and hypothetical example of such cooperativity would be if there were a gene causing blindness in the left eye and another gene causing blindness in the right eye. Possessing one gene would only mildly impair an individual's ability to reproduce, but possessing both would cause complete blindness and might well prevent the individual from reproducing at all. A milder, more realistic example might be a cooperative interaction between a cancer-promoting gene and another gene—say, the gene for albinism—that greatly increased the incidence of skin cancer in individuals carrying both genes compared with those carrying either gene alone. If, as seems likely, some degree of cooperativity is a general feature of harmful mutations, then individuals carrying more than a certain number of mutations would be very unlikely to survive long enough to reproduce. Once these individuals (the "losers") are out of the picture, the remaining individuals who carry fewer mutations (the "winners") are free to reproduce among themselves. If they do so sexually they mix their genes, and because of this mixture they produce a next generation with a wide diversity in the numbers of mutations possessed by each individual; that is, this generation has potential winners and losers just like the previous one. But if they reproduce *asexually,* the offspring will have a more uniform number of mutations per individual than the previous generation, because the extreme cases (the losers) in the previous generation never reproduced. This creates a problem: *some* fraction of the progeny are not going to be able to reproduce anyway, if the overall population size is limited, so now individuals who are closer to average in their number of mutations will have to be weeded out. In other words, even though the weeding-out process eliminates the same number of individuals, it cannot eliminate as many mutations from the asexually produced offspring as from the sexually produced offspring.

The Russian biologist and mathematician Alexei Kondrashov was able to show that, with plausible values for the mutation rate and the degree of cooperativity among harmful mutations, a female who reproduces sexually is indeed at an advantage over a female who reproduces asexually. Thus the genes for sexual reproduction will be maintained in the population.

This view of sex is almost the opposite of the traditional view. Traditionally, sex was thought of as a mechanism for generating exceptionally fit individuals. Kondrashov sees it as a mechanism for generating exceptionally *unfit* individuals: "runts" in other words, that will rapidly die and take a disproportionate share of their parents' harmful mutations with them.

There is certainly no agreement at the moment as to which of these theories, if any, are closest to the truth. Most likely the issue will eventually be resolved experimentally, that is, by directly observing the effects of artificial selection pressure on sexual and asexual varieties of small, rapidly propagating organisms.

What about the dandelions and asexual lizards? If sexual reproduction is generally beneficial as suggested by the arguments presented above, how do these species get along without it? Although there is no clear answer to this question, it is probable that these species were originally sexual and gave up sexual reproduction comparatively recently. The asexual lizards, for example, still go through the motions of sex; they just don't actually fertilize each other. Once the sexual individuals were eliminated (by circumstances we do not understand), the asexual individuals were no longer exposed to competition from them and therefore persisted. But in the long run Muller's ratchet may spell their doom.

So much for the possible reasons for the existence of sexual reproduction. But one can ask equivalent questions about all the details of sex. Why do the two sexes differ from each other in their anatomy and their behavior? What is the significance of courtship and mating rituals? Why are some species monogamous, others promiscuous? Why do some species (such as bees) contain a large proportion of sterile individuals? What is the ultimate cause of parental care, of sibling rivalry, and, for that matter, of human love and altruism? The attempt to answer such questions in terms of evolutionary theory constitutes the field of *sociobiology*. It is worth delving briefly into this field as a prelude to tackling the brain's role in sex.

First, why do the two sexes differ from each other? In the remote past there was probably not much difference between them. Not in the human past, that is, but among our unicellular ancestors many hundreds of millions of years ago. At that time the reproductive forms of organisms (the *gametes*) were probably all roughly similar in size and appearance. To reproduce sexually, they simply fused and combined their genes. But under natural selection these gametes gradually developed into two types: one (the female) became larger, while the other (the male) became smaller. This type of selection is called *disruptive,* because it breaks a single distribution (of sizes in this case) into two distributions.

The reason for disruptive selection for gamete size is believed to be as follows. In the original population some individuals would, by chance, have had genes causing them to be relatively small or relatively large. Those at the large end had an advantage, in that they contained more nutritive material for producing offspring, so these large individuals would tend to increase in number. But those at the small end also had an advantage, in that they could be produced more rapidly and with fewer nutrients. Admittedly, they contained less material to nurture offspring, but that would not matter too much if they mated with the large individuals and so took advantage of their mates' ample stores of nutrients. So the small individuals would also be favored and would increase in number too. Only the individuals of average size would have no special advantage and would gradually be eliminated, leaving separate populations of large (female) and small (male) gametes.

Eons have passed, and organisms have become vastly more complex, but the two sexes and their characteristic differences remain the same. Among vertebrates, the female gamete (the ovum or unfertilized egg) is vastly larger than the male gamete (the sperm). Since females invest so much in producing eggs, they are trapped in a nurturing role. They must do everything possible to ensure that their ovum is not wasted, because it will be so expensive to produce another. Eventually (in reptiles, birds, and mammals) the ovum is retained within the female's body, so that fertilization requires *copulation* between male and female. In mammals the developing embryo or embryos remain in the uterus for a prolonged period of fetal development, their needs supplied completely by the mother. This is a huge investment on the mother's part, not only because of the nutrients that need to be supplied but also because of the sacrifice of time that could have been spent producing more offspring. No wonder then that females are the ones that produce milk and nurse their young, and in fact generally take a greater role in helping their offspring survive in the world. The male can leave it all to the female, confident that she cannot afford to neglect her (and his) offspring.

Apparently, as we have discussed earlier, females cannot dispense with males entirely, because sexual reproduction produces offspring that are on average fitter than those that could be produced without sex. Still, from the female's point of view the male is little more than a parasite who takes advantage of her dedication to reproduction.

In most species, roughly equal numbers of males and females are produced. This may seem like the natural and best arrangement. But from the point of view of the well-being of the species as a whole, it would generally be better to produce an excess of females. This is because a small number of males can fertilize a much larger number of females; therefore most males are simply consuming valuable resources that could have gone toward producing females and their offspring. The fact that equal numbers of males and females are produced illustrates again the principle that natural selection operates at the level of the individual and the individual's genes, not at the level of the entire species. If less than 50% of the population were male, then males, on average, would have more than one female to fertilize, and thus they would have more offspring than females. In this case, producing males would be a better investment than producing females, so genes causing females to produce an excess of males would be favored. As a consequence, the overall sex ratio would soon return to 50:50.

Although evolution, as outlined above, has tended to make females the exploited sex, the situation changes somewhat when one realizes that females, through their *behavior,* can at least partially redress the balance. Because a few males can fertilize many females, a female has more of a choice about who she mates with than does a male. ("Choice" is a figure of speech: I don't mean that conscious processes are necessarily involved, but simply that there are generally a number of males with whom she could mate with equally little expense of time and effort.) Obviously, genes will be favored that cause her to make this choice in a way that benefits her reproductive success. Such behavior may consist of simply choosing the largest male, or the one who has proved himself the strongest by defeating in single combat every other male in the vicinity. But she can also choose in such a way as to increase the male's investment in their offspring. For example, a female bowerbird will only mate with a male that has devoted a huge amount of time and effort to constructing a gigantic, elaborate, and totally useless bower. The females of many species require the males to provide a large amount of food or to construct a nest as a condition for mating. If the male has made large investments of some kind prior to mating, he will be more likely to take an interest in the well-being of the young: it is just too expensive to abandon the family and start over. Of course, the female cannot take this strategy too far, otherwise other, less demanding females will supplant her. Still, there is a basic asymmetry in the situation, since a female can be pretty confident that she will be impregnated by *some* male, while a male, exposed as he is to cutthroat competition from his fellow males, risks never impregnating *any* female. This asymmetry gives the individual female leverage to make considerable demands on the male. In fact, it can have the result that the male and female devote roughly equal effort to parental care. In a few cases, indeed, it is the male who is left holding the baby while the female goes off in seach of new partners.

One of the major achievements of sociobiology has been the realization of the great influence that *kinship* has on behavior, including sexual behavior. Genes generally produce behavior that favors the individual's own survival and reproduction. However, if a particular gene is carried by a certain individual, it may also be carried by that individual's close relatives, because close relatives share many genes. Therefore, from the point of view of the survival of the genes, it may make sense to promote behavior that favors the reproductive success of close relatives, even at some cost to oneself. Charles Darwin was aware of this possibility, and it was followed up by R. A. Fisher and J. B. S. Haldane. The most detailed exploration of this theme, however, came in the 1960s when William Hamilton, then a graduate student at the University of London, put the theory of *kin selection* on an explicit quantitative footing.

The fundamental idea is simple. Although there is a baseline of genes that are shared by most or all members of a population, there are also a large number of genes that vary between individuals. Identical twins will of course have all these genes in common. Nonidentical twins and regular siblings have (on average) half of these genes in common. A parent and child also share half their genes. Half-siblings share (on average) a quarter of their genes, cousins one-eighth, and so on. According to the theory of kin selection, an individual will help a sibling if the benefit to that sibling is more than twice the cost to him- or herself. Similarly, an individual will help a cousin if the benefit to the cousin is more than eight times the cost to him- or herself. In other words, genes for altruistic behavior toward relatives are selected in evolution to the extent that the benefit to the recipient, *devalued by the degree of relatedness,* outweighs the cost to the individual who performs the altruistic act.

In practice, other important factors have to be taken into account. Generally animals (including humans) can not be sure about relationships. You can only be completely sure that you are related to yourself. A mother can be fairly sure who her offspring are (though even she can be mistaken—cuckoos stake their survival on that). A father can be less sure of whether the children in the family are really his, and the relationship between siblings is often uncertain. So, although there exist many mechanisms in the animal world for recognizing kin, there will be a tendency for individuals to favor themselves and their close relatives even more than suggested by the relationship outlined above, because of the decreasing certainty of relatedness that goes along with the decrease in relatedness itself.

It's no news that humans generally take kinship into account when helping others, especially when the help is given with little prospect of a return of the favor. Animals behave the same way. Much social behavior in animals is readily explicable by the rules of kin selection. Parents devote themselves altruistically to the care of their own offspring, but generally neglect, harass, or even kill unrelated offspring. Many animals give alarm calls in the presence of a predator, even though giving the call increases the risk that they themselves will be the predator's next meal, but careful observation has shown that such calls are almost always sounded by animals whose close relatives are nearby, and not by animals that are among unrelated individuals. Many animals sacrifice their own prospects of reproduction, either temporarily or permanently, to aid the reproduction of their relatives. Male lions, for example, operate in coalitions of several closely related animals, but one or two of these males do the lion's share of the mating; the others are repaid for their time and effort by the birth of nephews and nieces. The extreme cases are the worker ants and bees, females that forego all sex and instead toil unceasingly to aid their queen in her nonstop orgy of reproduction. It turns out that, due to a peculiarity of genetics in these species, workers are more closely related to the queen's offspring than to any offspring they might have had themselves. The close relatedness and the close cooperation are undoubtedly connected.

These considerations of kinship can lead to sexual behavior that is not what it seems. Take the following behavior observed by Sarah Hrdy among langur monkeys. Male langurs that seize the dominant position in a troop sometimes attempt to kill all nursing infants, as well as infants that are born up to several months after the takeover, since these infants were fathered by the previous dominant male. Killing these infants benefits the new leader because the mothers will rapidly become sexually receptive again, mate with him, and produce his offspring. The mothers, on the other hand, will do everything to prevent the infanticide, since from their point of view it is a sheer loss of investment: offspring sired by the new male are no more closely related to themselves than offspring sired by the previous male. Some females, pregnant by the previous male, come into a false heat—that is, they show every sign of sexual receptivity and allow the new male to mate with them, even though, being pregnant, they can neither ovulate nor conceive. Such behavior is highly unusual among animals other than humans: sexual receptivity is generally closely tied to ovulation. The point of this behavior, however, is revealed much later when the infant is born. The new male makes no attempt to kill the infant, but instead treats it as if it were his own. To put a conscious spin on it, the female, by mating with the new male while already pregnant, fools him into thinking he is the father of the infant that is born months later.

A naive person who had stumbled on this pair mating in the woods would undoubtedly have seen it as just another example of two animals cooperating amicably in the task of perpetuating their species. Only with many months of patient observation was it clear that the motives of the two animals were in radical opposition: one trying to sire young, the other trying to protect young already sired by another father.

Of course, we do not have to ascribe conscious thought to this behavior, either on the part of the gullible male or the devious female. Their genes see to it one way or another that they behave the way they do. Similarly, we do not know when in human evolution people first became

conscious of the causal connection between sexual intercourse and pregnancy; but it is not a crucial piece of information, because long before
then people were behaving *as if* they understood the connection. In sex,
as in so many other fields of action, consciousness may serve as much
to rationalize instinctive behavior as to provide its real motivation.

3

For a Woman Wert Thou First Created

The Biology of Sexual Development

In the previous chapter I outlined some ideas that biologists have put forward concerning the evolution of sex and sexual behavior. The message was basically this, that in matters concerning sex nothing can be taken at face value. Only careful observations, explicit theories, and experiments that test them can give us any confidence that we understand what is going on. Provisionally, though, we can say that sex and sexual behavior very probably evolved by natural selection acting at the level of the individual, that sexual reproduction was probably selected over asexual reproduction because, by providing for increased individual variability, it produces offspring that are on average fitter than those that could be produced asexually, and that much behavior, both sexual and nonsexual, can be explained in terms of selection for traits that favor the propagation of the individual's genes, either through that individual's own offspring or through the offspring of relatives.

I will return to human sexual behavior and its causes later. In this chapter I review what is known about the biological mechanisms that cause individuals to develop as male or female.

In humans, as in all mammals, sex is determined genetically. This is not true for all organisms. In alligators, for example, the sex of the offspring is determined by the temperature at which the eggs are incubated. Many organisms, especially plants, carry both sexes simultaneously, and others, such as certain fish, can change from one sex to the other. But in mammals it is a matter of what genes you inherit from your parents—specifically, what genes you inherit from your *father*.

The understanding of heredity and its chemical basis began with the realization, by the nineteenth-century German anatomist Haeckel, that the material responsible for heredity (a material we now know to be DNA) was located in the *nuclei* of cells, not in the cytoplasm. Meanwhile, Gregor Mendel deduced from plant-breeding experiments that there were discrete units of heredity—genes—whose passage from generation to generation obeyed simple laws. Further breeding work done in both plants and animals showed that some genes tend to be inherited together, and the pattern of this common inheritance (linkage) suggested that the genes were joined to each other in a consistent serial order. It later became clear that genes are located on the *chromosomes,* rodlike structures within the nuclei that become visible just prior to cell division, and that the degree of linkage between two genes is an expression of how close they are to each other along the chromosome.

By squashing some dividing cells (say, a sample scraped off the lining of the mouth), the chromosomes can be spread apart from one another, making them easier to examine and count. Except for sperm and ova (the gametes), the nuclei of human cells contain 46 chromosomes each. These 46 actually consist of 23 matched pairs. The two members of each pair are identical to each other in size and appearance, and they carry sets of corresponding, but not necessarily identical, genes. For example, at one location on a certain pair of chromosomes there is a gene that influences eye color. Both chromosomes possess such a gene at this particular location, but they may differ: one chromosome may carry a gene specifying blue eye color, the other may have a gene for brown eye color. If both genes say "blue" then your eyes will be blue, and if both say "brown" your eyes will be brown. But if one gene says "blue" and one says "brown" then your eyes will be brown: the brown gene dominates the blue one.

One pair of chromosomes, the *sex chromosomes,* is different from the other 22 pairs (the *autosomes*). In women, both sex chromosomes are long and closely resemble each other. These are called X chromosomes. In men, however, one member of the pair is long (X) and the other is very short (Y). What sex you are is determined by a gene situated on the Y chromosome. The gene is named *testis-determining factor* or *TDF* (the name suggests something about how this gene works, which we will get to later). If you have a Y chromosome you have the TDF gene and you develop as a male. If you do not have a Y chromosome you do not have this gene and you develop as a female.

When gametes are produced, there is a halving of the number of chromosomes. Sperm and ova contain only one member of each pair of chromosomes, for a total of 23 instead of 46. Which member of each pair is used depends on chance, and this is true both for the autosomes and the sex chromosomes. Thus a sperm will get either an X or a Y chromosome, because the male cells that produce it contain an X and a Y. An ovum, on the other hand, will always get an X, since the cells that produce it, being female, contain two X's. At fertilization the chromosomes of both gametes meet up to restore the full complement of 46 chromosomes. So, if the sperm that fertilized the ovum carried an X chromosome, the embryo will be XX and develop as a female; if the sperm contains a Y the embryo will be XY and will develop as a male.

Besides their role in sex, the sex chromosomes (particularly the X chromosome) carry other genes whose functions are quite different. For example, there are several genes on the X chromosome responsible for producing the light-sensitive pigments in the cone cells of our retinas, and another gene for one of the proteins concerned with bloodclotting. The fact that these genes are on the X chromosome means that their inheritance is *sex-linked* (specifically, that males inherit these genes from their mothers, not their fathers), but they are not functionally concerned with sex or sexual behavior in any way. Correspondingly, there are many genes on the autosomes that *are* concerned with sex, but their actions are controlled (via a long chain of causes and effects) by TDF.

Given the central importance of the TDF gene for sex differentiation, it is worth going into the history of its discovery and isolation. As soon as human chromosomes were characterized, attention focused on the Y chromosome as a likely site for a gene or genes determining sex, because it is the only chromosome that is present in one sex and not the other. However, there were other possibilities; for example, sex might be determined by a gene on the X chromosome, but the gene only works when present in two copies. Thus, if you have two X chromosomes you develop as a female, if you have less than two, you develop as a male. Or it might be the *ratio* of the number of X chromosomes to the number of autosomes that is crucial in determining sex (as it is, in fact, in some insects). These different models make quite different predictions about the sex of individuals who have unusual numbers of sex chromosomes. According to the first model (maleness caused by presence of at least one

Y chromosome) individuals who are XY (the usual male pattern), Y, XXY, or XXYY will all develop as males, while individuals with XX (the usual female pattern), X, or XXX will all be female. The second model (femaleness caused by two XX's, maleness by default) predicts that individuals with the XXY or XXYY patterns will be female, while individuals with the X pattern will be male. In fact, individuals with some of these unusual patterns are occasionally born, and the results nearly always support the first model: an individual with at least one Y chromosome will be male, and an individual without at least one Y chromosome will be female. (However, all individuals have to have at least one X chromosome, not for purposes of sex determination but because of all the other vital genes that are on that chromosome.) Thus it seemed likely that there was a gene (or genes) causing maleness on the Y chromosome, and that individuals lacking this gene developed by default as females.

By studying the rare individuals who are missing parts of the Y chromosome, or who carry a fragment of the Y chromosome attached to another chromosome, geneticists gradually homed in on the location of the sex-determining gene. Finally, the zone was defined so precisely that molecular biologists could snip out that region of DNA and analyze it, looking for a coding sequence that might be the gene. In 1990 a team at the Medical Research Council, Mill Hill, London (led by Peter Goodfellow and Robin Lovell-Badge) announced the discovery of such a candidate sequence at the appropriate location on the human Y chromosome, as well as a similar sequence on the Y chromosome of the mouse. They went on to show (in the mouse) that just this sequence, artificially incorporated into the genome of an otherwise normal XX mouse embryo, could cause it to develop as a male instead of a female, and hence was very likely to be the sex-determining gene TDF. This experiment, reported in 1991, was a major landmark in the history of sex research: it has opened up the prospect of following in molecular detail the chain of causation that leads from our genes to our male and female bodies and brains.

The sex chromosomes present in the fertilized ovum are handed down through many generations of cell division to all the cells of the body. Thus every cell, whether in the liver, the muscles, or the brain, has information defining its own sex, which is the same as the sex of the entire organism. One might think, then, that the sex differences that exist between male and female muscles, male and female livers (yes, they are different), and male and female brains result from the complement of sex chromosomes contained by the cells in these tissues—XX or XY. In insects, it does indeed work this way: sex-determination is *cell-autonomous*. But in humans and all other mammals it works quite differently. The sex-determining gene TDF works only in one tissue, the developing *gonad,* to make it develop into a male gonad, or *testis.* Hence the name "testis-determining factor." If TDF is not present, the gonad develops as an *ovary.* All the other sex differences, in genitalia, body size, muscles, liver, brain, body chemistry, and behavior, come about by the influence of the testis or ovary on the remainder of the body, an influence which takes no account of the genetic sex of the body cells. Thus, if the gonads of an XX mouse embryo were removed sufficiently early in development and replaced with the gonads from an XY embryo, then that embryo would develop into a normal, happy male mouse, even though all the cells in its body, except for those in its testis, were genetically female.

In the human embryo, the early undifferentiated gonads appear at about one month of gestation. At this time they lie at the back of the abdominal cavity, near the developing kidneys. Curiously, none of the cells forming these primitive gonads are destined to become gametes (sperm or ova). Instead, they will form supporting cells and hormone-producing cells. The founders of the gamete lines originate at a quite distant location in the embryo, namely in the yolk sac, a temporary organ that, confusingly enough, does not contain yolk. These founder cells take on the form of amoebas and crawl through a jungle of tissues until they finally home in on the gonads, where they intermingle with the locally born population.

Where and when does the TDF gene act? Although the details are not yet worked out, a likely scenario runs something like this. A set of genes common to both sexes drives the initial development of the gonad. At some point prior to the morphological differention into testis or ovary, one of these genes in the supporting cells commands the TDF gene to be turned on. If the embryo is a male, the TDF gene is present and is accordingly turned on, that is, the protein that it codes for is synthesized. If the embryo is female, the TDF gene is absent and so the command falls on deaf ears.

Let us first follow the sequence of events that result if TDF is absent, namely, the female developmental pathway. In this case the supporting cells continue on an internally programmed path of development that causes them eventually to become the cells that surround the ova in the follicles of the mature ovary (so-called *granulosa cells*). The cells of the hormone-producing lineage also continue on their own preprogrammed path, and develop into *thecal* cells of the ovary. These cells later synthesize steroid hormones, but they do not produce significant amounts of hormones during prenatal life. The gamete cells begin the process of halving their chromosome number as required for fertilization, but this process (called *meiosis*) is arrested soon after it begins and is not completed until adulthood. Nevertheless, the gamete cells influence the formation of the ovary: they must be present and they must have the appropriate number of X chromosomes (namely two). If they have only one X chromosome (the so-called *Turner's syndrome*), they die during prenatal development, and the entire ovary atrophies as a consequence.

Because the developing ovary does not produce appreciable amounts of hormones, the rest of the body is pretty much left to its own devices. That is, each part develops according to its own intrinsic program. The intrinsic program is to produce a female body. Thus an embryonic structure called the *müllerian duct* develops into the oviducts (Fallopian tubes), uterus, and cervix, and the tissue around the primitive urogenital groove differentiates into the female external genitalia: clitoris, labia, and vagina. Many other parts of the body, including the brain, differentiate in the female direction. I will return to the issue of brain development later. For now, the important point is that in fetal development, the pathway taken in the *absence* of sex-specific hormones is the female pathway. Only later in life, particularly at puberty, does further female development depend on hormonal instructions.

If the TDF gene *is* present in the supporting cells of the undifferentiated gonad, the protein that it codes for is synthesized. Although this protein has not been isolated, Goodfellow and colleagues were able to deduce its amino-acid sequence from the known DNA sequence of the TDF gene. A part of the amino-acid sequence turned out to be very similar to sequences in some other proteins that are known to be able to bind to DNA and regulate the expression of genes. Hence it is a good possibility that TDF also turns on other genes, presumably those which are required for differentiation of the supporting cells into the definitive male type of supporting cells called *Sertoli cells*. These are the cells that, beginning at puberty, nurture the developing sperm. Right away in the embryo, however, they send a message (whose nature is unknown) to the nearby cells of the hormone-producing lineage, instructing them to become the type of cell that produces steroid hormones (so-called *Leydig cells*). In addition, the supporting cells send another message which prevents the formation of the female genital tract (oviducts, uterus, cervix, and part of the vagina) from its embryonic precursor, the müllerian duct. This message is known to be a protein hormone, named müllerian-inhibiting hormone (MIH).

The Leydig cells now have a field day. They synthesize and secrete *testosterone* and related steroids (collectively called *androgens,* or male-makers). These hormones enter the bloodstream and guide the development of the entire body in the male direction.

Before getting into how this happens, we need to know a bit more about steroids, since they will play a major role in the remainder of this book. Steroids are a broad class of compounds synthesized from cholesterol, the fatty substance which, in spite of its bad reputation as an artery-clogger, is actually a vital constituent of every cell in the body. The cholesterol molecule consists of four connected rings, each ring being made of five or six carbon atoms. The ring at one end carries a tail of eight carbon atoms. Steroids are cholesterol molecules without their tails: the amputation is performed by a specific enzyme that is present only in a few types of cells in the body, including Leydig cells in the testis, thecal cells in the ovary, and cells of the adrenal gland.

Although all steroid hormones have the same basic four-ring structure, there are differences in the details of the structure that radically influence the way the hormones act. For example, testosterone has an oxygen atom attached to one of the carbon atoms (the so-called number 3 carbon). Estradiol, a steroid that plays a major role in female development, has a hydroxyl group (an oxygen and a hydrogen atom) at this same place. Progesterone, a steroid hormone that plays a vital role in reproduction by preparing the uterus for pregnancy, resembles testosterone in having a oxygen atom attached to the number 3 carbon atom, but it has two additional carbon atoms attached to the other end of the molecule (at the number 17 carbon). And so on. These subtle differences among the various steroids are generated by specific converting enzymes, which again are present only in certain types of cells. For example, Leydig cells do not possess the enzyme *aromatase,* which converts testosterone to estradiol; therefore Leydig cells cannot synthesize or secrete estradiol. Converting enzymes are found not only in the cells that carry out the initial synthesis of steroids from cholesterol (such as the Leydig cells) but also in many other cell types throughout the body. For example, some brain cells do contain aromatase and therefore can turn testosterone into estradiol. Inherited abnormalities or deficiencies in these converting enzymes can have dramatic effects on sexual development.

Steroids, like cholesterol, are fatlike substances: they dissolve readily in other fats but are poorly soluble in water. This has several consequences. First, steroids can pass readily through cell membranes, because cell membranes are largely made of fat. In contrast, protein hormones such as insulin cannot enter cells unaided; they generally act only at their outside surfaces. Second, most of the steroids in the blood are not in solution, but loosely attached to blood proteins such as albumen. Third, steroid molecules, being largely out of solution, have a relatively long lifetime: they survive for hours in the body, while insulin molecules survive only for minutes. Thus, while insulin can regulate blood sugar levels on a minute-by-minute basis in response to food intake, exercise, and so on, the processes regulated by steroids are generally slower processes, such as those involved in growth.

Not all steroids are involved in sex. One group, the *corticosteroids,* play a variety of roles in regulating the body's metabolism and its response to stress. These steroids are produced largely by the adrenal gland. The sex steroids are given the group name *gonadal steroids,* since they originate largely in the gonads. Nevertheless, the adrenal glands do produce small amounts of sex steroids too, and these steroids are of some significance in human sexual behavior, as will be discussed later.

Steroids act in a variety of ways, but the action that concerns us most is their ability to control the activity of genes. This is the mechanism by which the gonads have such a profound influence on the rest of the body: they are able to turn genes on or off in cells of many different tissues, thus influencing growth processes and many other biochemical activities.

This effect of steroids on genes is not a direct one. They first must be recognized and bound by *receptor* molecules in the cells of the target tissues. These receptors are large, globular proteins which, somewhere on their surface, possess a concavity whose shape and chemical structure is precisely designed to accommodate (bind) a steroid molecule. Somewhere else on the receptor is another site whose shape and chemical structure is precisely designed to bind DNA. In some fashion that we do not understand in detail, the presence of a steroid molecule in its binding site influences the other binding site: without the steroid present, the receptor binds DNA poorly or not at all, but once the steroid is attached, the receptor binds DNA avidly. So the presence of the steroid in the cell is the trigger that causes the receptor to act on genes.

The whole point of steroid receptors lies in their *specificity.* Any single type of receptor will bind one type of steroid much better than any other. Thus androgen receptors bind testosterone and similar steroids (androgens), estrogen receptors bind estradiol and similar steroids (estrogens), and progestin receptors bind progesterone and similar steroids (progestins). The distribution of these types of receptors in tissues is highly diverse. For example, even within one tissue, the brain, some cells have androgen receptors, some have estrogen receptors, some have progestin receptors, some have a combination of receptors, and many have none.

The specificity of steroid receptors is also seen in their binding to DNA. Each type of receptor binds a particular sequence of DNA better than any other sequence. Certain genes possess the characteristic DNA sequences that are recognized by androgen receptors, certain genes have the sequences recognized by estrogen receptors, and many others have no sequences recognized by any steroid receptors.

Thus we begin to see how the gonads can have such diverse effects on the rest of the body. If a particular gene in a particular cell is to be activated by the gonads, the following conditions must be fulfilled: (1) that gene must possess the characteristic DNA sequence allowing it to be bound by a particular steroid receptor, (2) the gene must not have been inactivated by some other overriding process (such as occurs, for example, when large blocks of genes, useless for a particular tissue or cell type, are permanently switched off during development), (3) the particular steroid receptor must be present in that cell, and (4) the steroid itself must be present in sufficient concentration, which means either that it must be present at sufficient levels in the bloodstream, or that the cell must contain converting enzymes capable of creating it from some other steroid that *is* present in the blood. Because of all these possibilities and conditions, the gonads can bring about many different effects in different regions of the body, both during development and later during adult life. For example, the gonads can cause one group of brain cells to become more electrically active, another less active, and another to form a particular set of synaptic connections or synthesize a particular chemical. Steroids can even control whether brain cells live or die.

Testosterone is first detectable in the blood of male human fetuses at about 2 months of gestation. Thereafter, the concentration does not rise gradually and smoothly; rather it follows a roller-coaster course with major peaks and troughs at predictable times. The first peak is at about 14 weeks, when the concentration of testosterone in the blood reaches about the same level as during puberty. Then it sinks to low levels, only to rise again toward the end of gestation. It peaks for the second time at about 2 months after birth. By about 6 months after birth the testosterone level has again fallen to low levels (about one-tenth of the adult level), remaining low until puberty, when it rises for a third time.

What is the significance of these peaks and valleys? Ideally, one would approach this problem by removing the male fetus's own source of testosterone, replacing it with an artificial supply whose level could be controlled, and observing the effects on development of eliminating one of the peaks or changing its timing. Obviously, one cannot do such experiments on humans. Therefore, one does the experiments in animals and tries to extend the conclusions to humans by comparing developmental stages, as well as by taking advantage of whatever disturbances of sexual differentiation occur naturally or by accident in humans.

The three most significant areas of sexual differentiation involve the internal genitalia, the external genitalia, and the brain. As to the *internal genitalia,* I described above how the precursor of the female internal genitalia, the müllerian duct, is caused to regress and atrophy in male fetuses by the action of the müllerian-inhibiting hormone secreted by the testis. There is another embryonic structure, named the *wolffian duct,* which has the potential to develop into the male internal genitalia. The development of these structures from the wolffian duct requires the presence of testosterone, and it takes place roughly in synchrony with the first peak in the blood level of the hormone. In female fetuses, lacking testosterone, the wolffian duct regresses.

Note the quite different strategies used for the sexual differentiation of the gonads and the internal genitalia. The male and female gonads develop from a common precursor; for this reason it is extremely rare for an individual to be born with the gonads of both sexes, although it can happen if the individual is a mosaic, in other words, is constituted of a mixture of tissues of different chromosomal make-up. The male and female internal genitalia, on the other hand, arise from different precursors, the wolffian and müllerian ducts. To become a normal male the embryo has to both switch *off* the müllerian pathway (with MIH) and switch *on* the wolffian pathway (with testosterone). If MIH is absent or ineffective, but testosterone or other androgenic steroids are present, the embryo may end up with parts or all of the internal genitalia of both sexes. This would be an example of *intersexuality*.

The differentiation of the *external genitalia* follows the same strategy as the that of the gonads, that is, the male and female genitalia differentiate from a common precursor, the tissue around the *urogenital membrane*. In the absence of testosterone, parts of this tissue develop into the clitoris, the labia minora and the labia majora, while in the presence of testosterone these same regions develop into the glans of the penis, the shaft of the penis, and the scrotum. Thus it is not possible for an individual to be born with male *and* female external genitalia. It is possible, however, for an individual to have external genitalia *intermediate* between those of a male and female. This is another type of intersexuality.

Although both internal and external genitalia develop in the male direction under the influence of circulating testosterone, there are two significant differences. First, the two processes are partially separated in time. Much of the differentiation of the external genitalia takes place around 5 and 6 months of gestation, after the first peak in testosterone levels has passed. Because of this difference in timing, events can affect one process more than the other. A good example of this is the condition known as *congenital adrenal hyperplasia*. This genetic abnormality of the adrenal glands causes them to secrete much larger amounts of androgens than usual. In female fetuses these excess androgens are capable of having a masculinizing effect on development. Because the internal genitalia differentiate relatively early, before the adrenal glands become functional, they are not affected. But the differentiation of the external genitalia *is* affected: they are masculinized to a variable degree. It is believed that the brain, which differentiates relatively late, can also be partially masculinized by the excess levels of androgens. The evidence for this will be discussed in later chapters.

The second difference is that the tissues of the external genitalia, unlike those of the internal genitalia, contain a converting enzyme named *5-alpha-reductase,* which converts testosterone to another androgenic steroid, dihydrotestosterone. This steroid binds to the androgen receptor even more effectively than does testosterone. This is why the external genitalia can develop in the male direction even during a period when circulating testosterone is at low levels; dihydrotestosterone works at much lower concentrations than testosterone. Here again is the possibility for the development of an intersex: if a fetus is chromosomally male but lacks the converting enzyme, the internal genitalia will develop as those of a male, but the external genitalia will be insufficiently masculinized, either being female or intermediate between male and female. Later, at puberty, circulating androgens rise to levels at which the tissue of the external genitalia *can* respond, and the child appears to change sex from female to male. This is the *5-alpha-reductase–deficiency syndrome,* which will be discussed in more detail in chapter 13.

These various abnormalities of development illustrate the possible complications in producing an all-male or an all-female body. They also offer opportunities to assess the influence of various developmental factors, and conditions of rearing, on the individual's ultimate gender identity and sexual behavior. These experiments of nature will be discussed in later chapters.

To sum up this chapter, we have seen that an individual's sex is determined by a single gene, named TDF, that is located on the Y chromosome. This gene causes an individual to develop as a male. TDF works by causing the undifferentiated gonads to develop as male gonads or testes. The testes in turn influence the remainder of the body to develop in the male direction; this influence is exerted by hormones, chief among which is the sex steroid testosterone. Sex steroids work by binding to receptor molecules in the target tissues such as skin and brain. The receptors then influence the expression of genes in the target tissues that cause these tissues to develop in a male-typical fashion. In females, who lack a Y chromosome and its TDF gene, the gonads develop into ovaries.

The ovaries do not secrete significant levels of sex steroids during fetal life, and, in the absence of such steroids, the body develops in the female direction. Thus one can say that female development is the default pathway, the one that is followed in the absence of specific instructions to the contrary. At puberty, however, the ovaries do begin to secrete high levels of estrogens, and these cause the body to complete its differentiation as a female. In the male, puberty is marked by a large increase in the production of testosterone, which causes the body to complete its differentiation as a male. The influence of gonadal steroids during development will be discussed further in later chapters. First, though, we must turn our attention to the brain.

4

What's in the Brain that Ink May Character?

Some Basic Principles of Brain Organization

The mind is just the brain doing its job. But to do that job, the brain has a structure that is intricate almost beyond belief, and functions that are complex almost beyond comprehension.

Almost, but not quite! Much about the brain is unknown, and the unknown can be disconcerting, but what we *do* know gives us some reassurance. As far as we can tell, the brain operates by ordinary physical laws and uses logical methods to achieve sensible ends. What has been discovered so far suggests that, though it may take a long time, in due course we or our descendants will understand it completely.

Take the brain's vital statistics. It contains about 10 billion nerve cells (neurons) and 10 trillion connections between nerve cells (synapses). These are certainly intimidating numbers. At first blush, they suggest a pattern of connectivity so vast and rich as to accommodate essentially any mode of operation one could possibly dream up. But what if one divides the second number by the first, that is, calculates what is the average number of connections made by a single neuron? The answer is about one thousand. This number is interesting, because it is so much smaller than the total number of neurons. Thus, even if each one of the thousand connections made by each neuron were with a *different* neuron, still each neuron could only be connected with a tiny fraction (1 in 10 million) of all the neurons in the brain. In other words, as a network the brain is vastly *underconnected*.

There is a second major fact to know about the brain. The great majority of all the synapses in the brain are made between nearby neurons—say within a millimeter or two of each other. That is not to say there are no long-distance connections. Some neurons in the motor region of the cerebral cortex, for example, have outgoing fibers (*axons*) that extend right down the spinal cord to form synapses with the motor neurons there, and these in turn have long axons that pass out of the spinal cord and form synapses with muscles. This is an example of a long pathway, whose function is to allow our cerebral cortex to send rapid orders for the execution of voluntary movements. Similarly, there is another long pathway (the optic nerve) that conveys visual information from the eye to visual regions of the brain. Both these pathways are obviously of great functional importance. Still, numerically these long connections are the exception; most connections (probably well over 90%) are local.

Actually, it almost *has* to be this way. If connections were made between neurons without regard to how close they were, the extra wiring would so crowd and cram the skull as to leave no room for the neurons themselves, or else our heads would have to swell to such a point that we would need the strength of an Atlas just to carry it on our shoulders. Even worse, mental processes would be painfully slow as we waited for signals to shuttle to and fro across it.

So synaptic connections in the brain are sparse and they are predominantly local. Putting these two facts together, we can deduce a third: the neurons in each small region of the brain can have only extremely limited information about what is going on elsewhere. In fact, nothing is so ignorant as a brain cell. A pattern of impulses impinges on it from neighboring cells, and perhaps from a few distant cells, but it knows little about what the vast majority of cells in the brain are doing, nor indeed does it know the meaning of those signals it does receive. It simply carries out some simple transformation of the incoming signals—adding them together, for example. In that sense, the brain's brilliance almost escapes us, the more closely we analyze it, just as one might peer ever closer at a painting in the hope of understanding its beauty, only to come up against crude brushstrokes and blobs of color.

Yet these very features aid our understanding. Each small region of the brain contains assemblies of cells working on a common task, whether it be to control the motion of a finger, to analyze the patterns of light in an image, to store a memory, or to generate sexual drive. Ultimately, of course, these assemblies must all interact, and indeed one can trace pathways, through a series of synapses, from any region of the brain to any other. But still there is enough independence between different regions to make it reasonable to approach the brain by trying to establish the function of each small region in turn.

Nothing illustrates this regional specialization of the brain better than the effects of local damage, such as may be caused by a stroke. A large stroke may be lethal, of course, or may eliminate many aspects of brain function, simply on account of the extensive territory that has been destroyed. But small strokes (or deliberately placed lesions in experimental animals) can have effects that are almost uncanny in their specificity. Just within the visual system, for example, cases have been documented in which a stroke has selectively eliminated the patient's ability to perceive color, or to see things in motion, while all other visual functions remain unaffected. Such findings strongly suggest that the analysis of color, motion, and other attributes of vision is carried out in a series of highly specialized subregions within the visual portion of the brain, and the location of the damage tells us where these regions are.

Experiments involving electrical stimulation of the brain also support the notion of regional specialization. The opportunity to do such experiments in humans are few, of course. Still, they are sometimes done in the course of neurosurgical procedures, and the results are startling. Stimulation of a given point on the cerebral cortex can cause the patient to make a particular movement or to recall a particular scene. Stimulation experiments in animals have told us an immense amount about brain organization. The results are not always easy to interpret. If stimulating a certain point in a monkey's brain makes it reach out its left arm, for example, is that because this is the part of the brain that controls movements of the left arm, or is it because the stimulation made the monkey see a banana somewhere off to the left and it is trying to grab it? With sufficient ingenuity, however, one can dissect out the various possibilities; one could decide between the two possibilities just mentioned, for example, by seeing what effect the same stimulation has when the monkey has eaten its fill of bananas, or when its left arm is tied behind its back.

One of the most remarkable discoveries to come from stimulation experiments was the finding, by James Olds and Peter Milner in the 1950s, that there are regions in the brain whose stimulation appears to be highly rewarding to the animal. If a rat is given the opportunity to stimulate itself at these sites—for instance, by pressing a lever that causes a current pulse or sequence of pulses to be delivered at the electrode tip—the rat will press the lever continuously until exhausted, passing up real rewards such as food or drink in order to do so. Once the rat has learned what pressing the lever does, it will swim moats, jump hurdles, or cross electrified grids to reach it. A huge literature has grown up around this phenomenon, and there is still considerable disagreement about its exact meaning. But it does suggest that even such an abstract notion as pleasure might have a correlate in the activity of a small group of neurons. Certainly one would not be surprised if brain regions concerned with sex were connected with such a system!

Yet another important source of information about regional specialization within the brain is the recording of the electrical activity of neurons. Most information of this type has come from the use of fine-tipped microelectrodes inserted into the brains of experimental animals. Such electrodes can pick up the impulses generated by a single neuron located near the tip of the electrode. In a 20-year collaboration, David Hubel and Torsten Wiesel at Harvard Medical School used this method to probe the visual part of the cerebral cortex in cats and monkeys. They found that each neuron increases its rate of electrical activity in response to very precisely defined attributes of the visual scene—for example, to the motion of a slit of light of a particular size and orientation, located at a particular spot in the animal's field of view and moving in a particular direction. More interestingly for our purposes, they found that the properties of adjacent neurons were very similar, though not identical. For example, the best orientation of the stimulus might be vertical for one cell and slightly tilted from vertical for its neighbor. As the electrode moved from cell to cell, the attributes of the stimulus preferred by each successive cell would gradually change. Thus the principle of orderly grouping of cells with common functions seems to extend down to the finest level that can be studied, at least in some parts of the brain such as the visual cortex. Hubel and Wiesel made the point that keeping cells with similar functional properties together in this fashion serves to minimize the length of connections required to assemble the entire array. The same principle probably applies to the brain as a whole.

Unfortunately, microelectrode recordings are generally impractical in humans. What few studies have been done—hurriedly in the course of neurosurgical procedures—have told us little more than that there are no glaring differences between the activity patterns of human neurons and those of animals, as indeed one might have predicted. But there are other techniques that can tell us something about functional specialization in the human brain. One recently developed technique that seems especially promising is positron emission tomography, or PET scanning. In this procedure a simple compound such as water is labeled with a short-lived radioactive isotope (in the case of water it would be a radioactive isotope of oxygen) and injected into the bloodstream of a human subject. The subject is then required to do some task—to read, say, or to do mental arithmetic. While this task is going on, the distribution of the radioactive isotope within the brain is determined by an array of detectors ranged around the head.

The reason this technique yields information about neuronal activity is that there is a tight coupling between neuronal activity and blood flow. If the neurons in a small region of the brain increase their activity, blood flow to this region is increased to allow for the extra metabolic demands of the active neurons, and so the level of radioactivity in this region increases. The local increase in blood flow caused by, say, reading can be identified by comparing a scan performed while the subject is reading with a second scan done while the subject is doing nothing. Desperately crude though this method is, in comparison with microelectrode recording, it does at least let one see the big picture, and to see it in the normal, functioning human brain. For example, reading text and listening to the spoken word each causes the activation of several small regions in the cerebral cortex. Some of these regions differ between reading and listening; these are the lower centers, which are engaged in deciphering the sight or the sound of the words. Other regions are identical in the two situations; these are presumed to be higher centers that are engaged in linguistic analysis without regard to the particular modality by which the words were acquired. This technique has not yet been applied to the study of sex; perhaps researchers are waiting for the construction of machines big enough to accommodate two subjects at once!

Although the evidence for local specialization of function in the brain is overwhelming, one has to inject a note of caution. It is not entirely clear what one should understand by "specialization." A set of experiments on a certain brain region might lead one toward a conclusion like "This a center for playing the clarinet." But realistically, playing the clarinet is a highly elaborate behavior requiring motivation, memory, muscular coordination, sight, hearing and touch—even a sense of musicality if one is to do it well. It is not likely that one small part of the brain could do all of that. On the contrary, it is certainly distributed over many systems and circuits. Instead one should express a brain region's function in terms that neurons themselves might understand—something like "This is a center for taking such-and-such inputs and performing such-and-such a transformation on them." What this neural activity would mean for the person's actual behavior would depend on the chain of connections and transformations interposed between this region and the person's muscles.

If you slice into the brain and look at the cut surface, you will see two colors, white and pinkish-tan. The white regions are called, logically enough, *white matter.* These are the brain regions that contain nothing but axons. A well-known piece of white matter is the *corpus callosum,* the huge band of axons connecting the left and right hemispheres of the cerebral cortex. Nothing interesting happens in the white matter (it's just impulses traveling along wires), but damage to the white matter can be devastating, in the same way that a backhoe that slices through a buried telephone cable can paralyze an entire city.

The pinkish-tan regions are called (less logically) *gray matter,* and this is where all the action is. The gray matter contains all the cell bodies of the neurons, all their local processes, and all their synapses. Gray matter itself comes in two kinds: *cortical* and *nuclear* structures. Cortex is gray matter arranged in layers at the outside surface of the brain. The cerebral cortex is the largest example, so well known that it is sometimes simply referred to by the generic name cortex. The cerebellum, the structure that is tucked under the back of the cerebral cortex and attached to the stem of the brain, also has an extensive cortex over its surface. Characteristic of cortex is its highly repetitive structure: one piece of the cerebral cortex looks very much like another, although an expert can tell the difference. As for the cerebellar cortex, not even an expert can tell which region a particular sample comes from. This repetitiveness of structure immediately invites the speculation that cortical structures perform a similar task over and over again, not in time but in space. That is, different regions of the cerebral cortex might take different inputs—say, visual inputs to one and auditory inputs to the other—and subject these inputs to a roughly similar type of transformation. Indeed, there is some evidence that this is the case, even if we do not really grasp what the nature of this fundamental process is. When people refer to the brain as operating in a "massively parallel" fashion (and hold this up as a model for the next generation of supercomputers), they are usually thinking of the cortical type of organization.

The *nuclear* structures are generally located within the substance of the brain. Like galaxies of stars, these are aggregates of large numbers of neurons. Most of them are not organized in any obvious layered pattern. Each aggregate is called a nucleus; this meaning of the word has nothing to do with the nuclei of cells, or with the nuclei of atoms for that matter. Brain nuclei come in a great variety of sizes: the smallest might be about the size of a grain of sand and contain a few thousand cells, the largest might be the size of a nut and contain some tens of millions of cells. Each nucleus has a name, which may celebrate its discoverer ("Deiter's nucleus"), its shape ("lentiform nucleus"), its color ("red nucleus"), its position ("dorsomedial nucleus"), or any of a number of real or fancied attributes. Generally the one thing the name does not tell you is its function, since the names were assigned centuries ago by anatomists who had not the slightest inkling what the structures did. In many cases, we still do not know, but as a general rule it seems that most or all of the neurons in a nucleus share similar connections and have a similar function.

As galaxies come in clusters, so brain nuclei are often grouped into larger assemblies. The largest of these is the *thalamus,* a lemon-sized cluster of about twenty nuclei located at the center of the brain, well hidden from view. The nuclei of the thalamus are intimately connected in two-way fashion with the cerebral cortex; almost all the information destined for the cortex must first be processed in the thalamus. In some way that we only dimly understand, the thalamus plays an important role in controlling consciousness. It seems to do this both by determining what inputs are allowed to pass through to the cerebral cortex, and also by directly modulating the level of excitability of neurons in the cerebral cortex. You may remember that a couple of chapters ago I dismissed consciousness as largely irrelevant to human behavior. That may have been somewhat tongue-in-cheek, but still the fact is that the thalamus has only a bit part in the drama of sex.

Right beneath the thalamus, though, and forming the brain's soft underbelly, is another nuclear cluster that plays both leading man and leading lady. This is the *hypothalamus,* topic of the next chapter.

To summarize what I have said about the brain so far, this is an extraordinarily complex tissue, yet one that is organized according to certain simplifying principles. The units of brain function—nerve cells or neurons—are grouped into local assemblies, which may be cortical (layered) or nuclear (nonlayered) in organization. Within an assembly, neurons share many structural and chemical features in common, and have similar connections with other parts of the brain. Experiments involving destruction or artificial stimulation of these assemblies, or the recording of their electrical activity, have shown that each assembly, by performing a particular transformation of the signals reaching it, plays a discrete role in the perceptual or behavioral life of the organism.

5

The Womby Vaultage

A Visit to the Hypothalamus

People tend to stay away from the hypothalamus. Most brain scientists (including myself until recently) prefer the sunny expanses of the cerebral cortex to the dark, claustrophobic regions at the base of the brain. They think of the hypothalamus—though they would never admit this to you—as haunted by animal spirits and the ghosts of primal urges. They suspect that it houses, not the usual shiny hardware of cognition, but some witches' brew of slimy, pulsating neurons adrift in a broth of mind-altering chemicals. Let us descend to this underworld.

The first thing that strikes one about the hypothalamus is how small it is. Even though it plays a key role in sex, feeding, drinking, cardiovascular performance, control of body temperature, stress, emotional responses, growth, and many other functions, it occupies a mere level teaspoonful or so of brain tissue.

Flipping the brain on its back to inspect this dime-sized area, one can see several landmarks. First, toward the rear, are what look for all the world like a pair of miniature breasts protruding from the brain surface. In recognition of the resemblance, these are called the *mammillary bodies*. Ironically, this part of the hypothalamus has nothing to do with sex.

In front of the mammillary bodies is another, single bulge. Since it is in the midline it is named the *median eminence*. From the center of the median eminence a stalk-like structure, made up of axons and blood vessels, runs downward into a deep cavity excavated in the floor of the skull. In this cavity, about the size of a pea, sits the *pituitary gland*. The stalk connecting the hypothalamus with the pituitary gland is the route by which the nuclei in the hypothalamus control the secretory function of the gland.

In front of the stalk of the pituitary gland is yet another landmark. This is the X-shaped crossing of the left and right optic nerves, termed the *optic chiasm.* Although the chiasm is located on the surface of the hypothalamus, most of the axons in the optic nerves do not end here but instead pass upward to the thalamus. A few optic axons do terminate in the hypothalamus, however, in a nucleus situated immediately above the chiasm and appropriately named the *suprachiasmatic nucleus.* This nucleus is the central pacemaker for circadian rhythms, and the optic nerve axons that synapse here bring information about the intensity of ambient illumination—information that the suprachiasmatic nucleus uses to judge whether it is night or day.

The substance of the hypothalamus extends from these surface landmarks upward for a few millimeters, until it reaches the undersurface of the thalamus. The hypothalamic tissue (as well as the thalamus above it) is divided in the midline by a watery cleft, the *third ventricle;* hence the hypothalamus has symmetrical left and right halves. Each of the twenty or so nuclei in the hypothalamus are actually duplicated, one on the left and one on the right. As far as we know, the two members of each pair have the same structure, the same connections and the same function, so they are often casually referred to in the singular (as the suprachiasmatic *nucleus,* for example, rather than the two suprachiasmatic *nuclei*).

In many ways the hypothalamus resembles any other group of nuclei in the brain. For the most part its nuclei comprise conventional-looking neurons, which make numerous connections among themselves as well as receiving and sending some long-distance connections to other parts of the brain. But in some other respects the hypothalamus is quite unusual. First, much of the information that the hypothalamus receives does not come in the form of neuronal messages, but in the form of direct physical or chemical stimulation of the hypothalamus itself. For example, some neurons in some hypothalamic nuclei are directly sensitive to local temperature, and use this sensitivity as part of a mechanism for the regulation of body temperature. Others are sensitive to substances in the blood such as glucose or salt, and are involved in regulating the levels of these substances. Still others are sensitive to circulating hormones, among which are included gonadal steroids such as testosterone. This sensitivity is mediated by steroid receptors as described in chapter 3.

On the output side, the hypothalamus is also unusual. For sure, there are many hypothalamic neurons whose output is conventional, in the sense that their axons form synapses with other neurons, either nearby or in distant regions of the brain or spinal cord. Some of these are directly concerned with generating sexual behavior. In addition, though, there are other hypothalamic neurons whose function is to synthesize and secrete hormones. These are termed *neuroendocrine* cells by virtue of their intermediate character between conventional neurons and glandular cells. Some hypothalamic hormones have effects on distant targets in the body. One of these, *oxytocin,* is involved in orgasm, giving birth, and breast feeding, as will be described later. Most of them, however, work locally by controlling the release of a second set of hormones synthesized by the pituitary gland. The pituitary hormones include several that influence the gonads as well as other organs involved in reproduction such as the uterus and breasts. This two-step hormonal pathway is a major route by which the hypothalamus exerts its control over matters of sex and reproduction.

The structure of the hypothalamus may be studied in human brains obtained at autopsy, or in experimental animals that have been killed for this purpose. Typically, the brain is preserved and hardened in formaldehyde, then the hypothalamus is cut into thin slices or *histological sections,* each about 0.02 mm thick, with the aid of a microtome. The sections are mounted on slides and stained with dyes that color the neurons and hence make them visible under a microscope. In these sections, one can recognize the various nuclei of the hypothalamus on the basis of the appearance of the neurons forming them. As an example, a nucleus termed the *supraoptic nucleus* contains very large, densely staining, and closely packed neurons. These neurons synthesize oxytocin, the hormone mentioned above. Immediately next to the supraoptic nucleus is the *suprachiasmatic nucleus,* also mentioned above, whose neurons are very small, pale, and scattered. By themselves, however, such sections tell one little about the connections or functions of the structures that are visualized.

One method that has greatly increased the amount of information that can be obtained from histological sections is the use of antibodies to label compounds of interest. This procedure is known as *immunohistochemistry.* Let us say one wanted to know which neurons in the hypothalamus contained oxytocin. Antibodies to oxytocin are generated by immunizing a rabbit with purified oxytocin. The sections of the hypothalamus are then placed in a solution containing a small amount of the rabbit's serum (the component of the blood that is rich in antibodies), and the antibodies in the serum bind to the oxytocin in the neurons. The sections are then transferred to another solution that contains a substance capable of binding to the rabbit antibodies. This might be serum from an animal of another species (a goat, say) that had been immunized against rabbit antibodies. The antibodies in this secondary antiserum are "labeled" in some way prior to use. For example, they might be joined to molecules of a fluorescent dye. Thus the fluorescent dye molecules will themselves become attached (indirectly via the two sets of antibodies) to the oxytocin molecules in the sections. Viewed under a fluorescence microscope, the oxytocin-positive cells shine brightly against a dark background. It turns out that the supraoptic nucleus contains many oxytocin-positive cells. Immunohistochemistry has been used to localize hormones, neurotransmitters, receptors, and other substances to particular cell groups within the hypothalamus.

The synthesis of these various substances by neurons depends ultimately on the activity, or "expression," of the genes that code for them. Gene expression can be studied in tissue sections by an ingenious technique called *hybridization histochemistry*. The first step in the expression of a gene is the separation of the two strands of the double helix of DNA and the copying of one of the strands into RNA (ribonucleic acid). This so-called *messenger RNA* (mRNA) passes from the nucleus into the cytoplasm and acts as a template for the synthesis of proteins. If the nucleic acid sequence of the gene, or part of the gene, is known, it is possible to synthesize a radioactive nucleic acid (either DNA or RNA) whose sequence is complementary to the sequence of that particular mRNA, in other words, a chain that will wind up into a double helix with it (hybridize). Thus if the tissue section is incubated in a solution containing such a radioactive probe, the radioactivity accumulates in those cells that contain that particular type of mRNA. The radioactivity can then be detected by *autoradiography*, that is, by coating the section with a photographic emulsion, letting it sit in the dark for a few days while the radioactivity exposes the emulsion, and then developing it like a photograph. The result is a cluster of developed silver grains lying over the cell containing that mRNA. The beauty of this technique is that it allows one to directly measure changes in gene expression that occur in particular sets of neurons under the influence of external signals—for example, to monitor how the rise and fall of gonadal hormones during the menstrual or estrous cycle in turn influence the synthesis of brain hormones by various groups of hypothalamic neurons.

While on the subject of techniques, it is worth saying a word about how connections are traced in the brain. You might think that one could do this simply by dissecting the brain, or else by following an axon or a group of axons through a series of histological sections from the neuronal cell bodies where they originate to the terminals where they form synaptic contacts with other neurons. These were in fact the methods used by early neuranatomists, and they generally got it wrong. It's simply too much of a jungle in there—finding a particular axon in a section is like trying to find a particular piece of hay in a haystack.

Two major technical advances have given us the tools to trace neuronal connections in an accurate and detailed fashion. The first was a serendipitous discovery by the Italian neuroanatomist Camillo Golgi in the 1870s. He took a piece of brain tissue that had been soaked in a fixative solution containing potassium dichromate, and dropped it into another solution containing silver nitrate. As any chemist could have predicted, precipitates of highly insoluble silver chromate formed in the tissue. What was totally unexpected, however, was that the precipitates filled only a few neurons (maybe 1% of the total) but filled them and their axons completely. In the histological sections the metal-filled cells and their axons stood out brilliantly against an unstained background. Now the problem was reduced to finding a needle in a haystack, a relatively simple task. Most of what we know about local connections in the brain is derived from the use of Golgi's method. More recently, it has become possible to impale single neurons in the living brain with an extremely fine-tipped pipette and inject fluorescent dyes into them. This produces an image similar to that obtained with Golgi's method, but has the additional advantage that the electrical activity of the cell can be recorded through the same pipette. With this technique a direct correlation can be made between a neuron's form and its function.

Both these methods yield valuable information about local connections, but they are not very practical for studying long connections, that is, the connections between neurons lying in totally separate regions of the brain. For this task a quite different class of techniques has been developed. These techniques take advantage of the fact that neurons are constantly shipping substances up and down their axons, a phenomenon known as axonal transport. Many tracer substances, such as radioactively labeled amino acids, can hitch a free ride on these neuronal highways. Thus if one of these tracers is injected into a small region of the brain, then a few hours or days later it will be found in other brain regions that are connected to the region that was injected. This approach really took off in 1971 when it was discovered that the enzyme peroxidase, extracted from horseradish, was taken up by neurons and transported in this fashion. Although peroxidase is not itself visible in tissue sections, it can catalyze (promote) a histochemical reaction that leads to the deposit of colored substances at the sites where the enzyme is located. This discovery provided a method for tracing connections that was at once simple and exquisitely sensitive. Twenty years later, papers describing results obtained with this method, and others derived from it, are being published at the rate of several a week. Luckily, the brain is sufficiently complex to support this particular industry for years to come.

Of course, these tracer techniques cannot be applied to humans. Unless methods for studying connections noninvasively in the living brain are developed, we will remain largely dependent on information derived from experiments performed in animals. This is a major limitation, especially when one is interested in the circuitry underlying activities like sexual behavior, which differ markedly from one species to another.

The hypothalamus has been studied intensively with all these anatomical methods as well as with the functional methods discussed in the previous chapter (electrical recording, electrical stimulation, and observing the effects of localized damage). Many of the findings will be described in later chapters devoted to particular aspects of sexual behavior. A lot remains unknown, but what we know so far is enough to assure us that there is a remarkable specificity of form and function. Even though the hypothalamus does not have the highly repetitive, almost crystalline architecture of structures like the visual cortex, there is nothing vague or diffuse—let alone slimy—about it. The hypothalamus consists of sets of neurons, each reliably indentifiable on the basis of size, shape, position, and chemical constituents, each with a particular pattern of synaptic connections with other sets of neurons, and each contributing a definable operation to a complex, cooperative endeavor. It is this specificity that makes it possible to search for the neuronal basis for differences between individuals in sexual behavior.

6

The Beast with Two Backs
The Elements of Sexual Intercourse

This chapter is devoted primarily to garden-variety, heterosexual, penile-vaginal intercourse, also known as coitus, copulation, or what you will. It is a suitable place to begin, since it is an unequivocally sexual behavior, and yet so simple, one hardly needs a brain to do it. Later, we will go on to what leads up to intercourse, what may follow it, and variations on it.

The reason why one hardly needs a brain is that many of the neuronal circuits that mediate coitus lie not in the brain but in the spinal cord. Copulation is a series of reflexes: one thing leads to another. Nevertheless the brain, especially the hypothalamus, does control and modulate these reflexes, and the subjective experiences connected with coitus, especially the experience of orgasm, obviously require a brain.

The basic components of coitus in humans are (1) erection of the penis; (2) engorgement of the walls of the vagina and the labia majora, lubrication of the vagina by glandular secretions and transudation, and erection of the clitoris; (3) insertion of the penis into the vagina (intromission); (4) pelvic thrusting by one or both partners; (5) elevation of the uterus, with a consequent forward and upward rotation of the mouth of the cervix; (6) ejaculation of semen into the vagina; and (7) orgasm, the intensely pleasurable sense of climax and release, often accompanied by increases in heart rate, flushing of the skin, muscle spasms, and involuntary vocalizations.

The behavioral patterns of coitus are much less sex-differentiated in humans than in animals. In most mammals the male approaches the female from the rear. This necessitates radically different postures on the part of the male and the female. In rats, for example, the female flexes her back in an U-shape (*lordosis*), thus exposing her genital area for intromission by the male, who mounts her, grasps her back, and thrusts with his pelvic muscles. Lordosis and mounting are readily distinguishable "female-typical" and "male-typical" motor patterns. In humans, on the other hand, the overt motor patterns of coitus are less clearly differentiated between the sexes, so that one would not necessarily expect major differences in the neuronal systems that produce these patterns.

There are some differences, however, and these are of considerable interest from the standpoint of the nervous system and its development. Among them is a difference related to erection. Both the male penis and the female clitoris are erectile, and both become erect reflexively in response to local mechanical stimulation as well as to psychogenic causes (i.e., sexually arousing thoughts, proximity of sexual partner, etc.). In both cases, erection is basically a hemodynamic phenomenon—that is, it results from an increase of arterial blood flow into the organ and a decrease of venous drainage from it. But the penis, as well as possessing larger reservoirs for engorgement with blood, also contains the attachments of two long muscles with even longer names: ischiocavernosus and bulbocavernosus. These muscles, besides making the erect penis moveable, participate in erection, especially the final, extreme phase of erection that precedes ejaculation, and they also participate in ejaculation itself. In women the ischiocavernosus is much smaller than in men, and the bulbocavernosus forms circular, constrictive fibers around the vagina. Correspondingly, the spinal cord of men contains a larger number of the motor neurons that innervate these muscles than are found in women.

This kind of anatomical difference between the sexes is known as a *sexual dimorphism.* It is interesting to find such a difference in the spinal cord, that is, at a very low level of the nervous system. Marc Breedlove and Arthur Arnold at the University of California, Berkeley, have made a special study of how this dimorphism arises during development. They used rats and mice, in which the sex difference is even more marked than in humans.

Breedlove and colleagues found that, early in development, both the muscles and the motor neurons are present equally in both sexes. In female pups, the muscles and the motor neurons regress and die, while in males they survive and grow. The difference is caused by hormones—specifically, by the presence of circulating testosterone in the male pups and its absence in females. There is a particular *critical period* during which testosterone must be present in adequate levels for the muscles and neurons to survive. In rats this period extends from a few days before birth till about 5 days after birth. Exposure of female rats to testosterone during this period (by injection of testosterone into the pregnant mother or into the newborn pups), masculinizes the muscles and the spinal motor neurons, while blocking of the effects of testosterone in male rats during this same period (by administration of an artificial androgen-blocking drug or by castration) causes the muscles and neurons to atrophy and die, leaving the female pattern.

How does testosterone act to cause survival of the spinal motor neurons? One possibility is that the hormone acts directly on the neurons themselves, binding to androgen receptors that in turn perhaps activate genes required for the neurons' survival. But another possibility is that the hormone acts only on the muscles, promoting their survival, and that the death of motor neurons in females is an indirect effect, resulting from the death of the muscles. This possibility is a real one, because it is known from other experiments that motor neurons generally die if their target muscles are destroyed. In fact, it appears that this second explanation is the correct one, because during the critical period only the muscles, and not the neurons, possess detectable levels of androgen receptors. Breedlove confirmed this by making genetically engineered mice in which the neurons carried a mutation that rendered them permanently incapable of synthesizing functional androgen receptors, while the muscles carried normal receptors. In these mice, just as in normal mice, the presence of testosterone during the critical period caused the neurons to survive. This strongly supported the notion that the death or survival of the the neurons is secondary to the death or survival of the muscles that they innervate.

Nevertheless, there is also a direct effect of testosterone on the motor neurons, as might be expected from the fact that they do possess androgen receptors later in life: although testosterone does not directly affect their survival, it does influence their growth and the formation of synapses. This type of effect will be discussed later in connection with the sexual differentiation of the hypothalamus.

Returning to the mechanics of copulation, let us take a look at lordosis, the crouching, raised-rump posture adopted by females of many species when mounted by males. Lordosis is one of the most intensively studied of all sexual behaviors; Donald Pfaff and other scientists at the Rockefeller University have made especially important contributions in this area. Lordosis is not a standard component of sexual intercourse in humans, although even a cursory perusal of "adult" magazines will convince you that humans (of both sexes) do have it in their repertoire.

Lordosis in rats is basically a reflex, like the knee-jerk. The sensory trigger for the reflex is touching or grasping of the skin of the flank or rump. In nature this would usually be done by the male as he begins to mount the female. The response is an activation of motor neurons that innervate the deep longitudinal muscles of the back, which leads to inverse arching of the spine. Unlike the ischiocavernosus and bulbocavernosus muscles, the muscles involved in lordosis are general-purpose muscles with a role in many nonsexual behaviors such as locomotion. Thus the muscles themselves, and the spinal motor neurons that innervate them, are similar in the two sexes.

The lordosis reflex differs from the knee-jerk in two ways. First, its circuitry is not contained entirely within the spinal cord, since in rats at least it disappears after the spinal cord is surgically separated from the brain (the knee-jerk actually becomes stronger after this operation). Second, the lordosis reflex is overlaid with several layers of control from higher centers in the brain. The activity of these control circuits has the effect that the reflex is elicited most readily in the most appropriate circumstances, namely, at the right time in the estrous cycle (around the time of ovulation), and in the presence of a partner of the right species and sex.

The estrous (or menstrual) cycle will not be discussed in detail in this book. Suffice it to say that the female rat's sexual receptivity, and the ease with which the lordosis reflex can be elicited, peak around the time of ovulation. These behavioral changes are controlled by the cyclical changes in circulating levels of the steroid hormones secreted by the ovary—estrogens and progestins. If a rat's ovaries are removed, sexual behavior, including the lordosis reflex, rapidly disappears but can be restored by administration of these hormones. The main site of action of the hormones in facilitating the reflex is in the hypothalamus, primarily in one nucleus within the hypothalamus named the *ventromedial nucleus,* which plays a central role in the generation of female-typical behavior. The function of this nucleus, and the manner in which it is influenced by steroids, will be taken up in chapter 9.

Ejaculation and orgasm—the climax of sexual excitement—are brought about by a complex interaction of neuronal and hormonal processes, which are still incompletely understood. Immediately preceding ejaculation in men, seminal fluid and the glandular secretions of the prostate are emitted into the back of the urethra. This emission occurs under the influence of a barrage of activity in the sympathetic nervous system, a set of nerve fibers that originates in ganglia near the spinal cord and that uses adrenalin as a neurotransmitter. Other effects of sympathetic activity, such as an increase in heart rate and blood pressure, occur at the same time. Emission is not a necessary precursor to orgasm, however; some men who are taking drugs that block the action of the sympathetic nervous system achieve orgasm without emitting any seminal fluid. Furthermore, although emission is accompanied by a strong sense of the inevitability of ejaculation, the sudden curbing of sexual activity or excitement can prevent ejaculation even at this late point; in this case semen flows passively from the urethra as it does during nocturnal emissions ("wet dreams").

Ejaculation is accomplished by the contraction of the bulbocavernosus and ischiocavernosus muscles, as well as of the muscular walls of the urethra itself. The semen is ejected violently against the mouth of the cervix, or against whatever barrier human ingenuity has placed in its way. Ejaculation is accompanied by the intense emotional sense of climax and release known as orgasm, and often by involuntary cries and muscle spasms throughout the body.

A recently discovered feature of orgasm is that it is accompanied by a massive release of the hormone oxytocin from the pituitary gland. Oxytocin is synthesized by neurons in two nuclei of the hypothalamus, the supraoptic and paraventricular nuclei. The hormone is not released into the bloodstream in the hypothalamus itself; instead, it is transported down the axons of the neurons to their terminals in the pituitary gland, which are located close to blood vessels. The sudden release of the hormone is probably caused by a burst of impulses generated by the same neurons; the impulses, reaching the axon terminals, cause release of the hormone in the same manner that neurotransmitters are released by more conventional neurons.

Michael Murphy and his colleagues at the Institute of Psychiatry in London showed that the release of oxytocin at ejaculation could be completely prevented by intravenous infusion of the drug naloxone. Naloxone is a specific antagonist of the action of opiate drugs and of the natural opiate-like substances (endorphins) that are present within the brain. Thus Murphy's finding suggests that the release of oxytocin at orgasm is under the control of the endorphin system, which is believed to be centrally involved in arousal and pleasure. Interestingly, the naloxone infusions had no effect of the men's ability to achieve sexual arousal, erection, and ejaculation, or on their heart rate or blood pressure during sexual activity. But the subjects did report that they had less pleasurable orgasms during the naloxone infusion than during infusion of an inactive substance (a placebo). Does this mean that the oxytocin surge is responsible for the subjective pleasure of orgasm? Possibly so, but it is also possible that naloxone has its effect by blocking pleasure-causing circuits elsewhere in the brain, and that the effect on oxytocin release is coincidental or secondary. More research is needed before one could confidently describe orgasm as an "oxytocin high."

Orgasm in men is followed by detumescence of the penis and return of heart rate, etc. to baseline values. For at least a few minutes after orgasm, penile erection and ejaculation are impossible; this is the *refractory period.* It is unclear what causes this unresponsiveness, but the length of the period is influenced by psychological factors. In rats, for example, a male that has just ejaculated will mount a new female more speedily than he will remount the same female with whom he has just copulated. This is the so-called *Coolidge effect,* named after President Calvin Coolidge. Here is the reason for the name, as recounted in Philip Groves and George Rebec's excellent *Introduction to Biological Psychology:*

Legend has it that President Coolidge and his wife were visiting a chicken farm in the Midwest when his wife wanted to know if just one rooster kept all the hens sexually active. When a farmer confirmed that this was true, Mrs. Coolidge wanted her husband to know about it. After the farmer told Mr. Coolidge, the president asked the farmer to remind Mrs. Coolidge of one important fact: The rooster takes on a different hen each time.

Sexual climax in women and men is remarkably similar. The physiological manifestations and the subjective quality of orgasm seem to be indistinguishable in the two sexes. Furthermore, many women experience a spurt of glandular fluid at the time of orgasm. This "female ejaculation" has been the subject of considerable controversy: some people who have studied the phenomenon (such as Masters and Johnson) believed that it was rare, and that the fluid was generally urine; that is, the "ejaculation" was nothing more than a brief urinary incontinence associated with the stress of sexual climax. More recent studies suggest that the fluid derives from glands near the urethra that may be homologous to the male prostate gland. A large survey of women conducted by Carol Anderson Darling and colleagues revealed that female ejaculation is quite common: about 40% of women reported having experienced it. Ejaculation occurred more commonly with orgasms that followed stimulation of the sensitive area within the vagina (the Grafenberg spot) than with orgasms caused by stimulation of the clitoris. (It is somewhat ironic that the replies from lesbian women, who have the best opportunity to observe these phenomema, were excluded from the study.)

The main difference between male and female orgasm is that in women it is not necessarily followed by a refractory period. Many women (over 40% in another survey by Darling and colleagues) frequently experience two or more orgasms in a row without descending from the plateau phase of sexual arousal. It is very possible that most women can experience multiple orgasms, but do not do so for lack of experimentation or because of psychological or social inhibition. In fact, the majority of women in the Darling survey who generally experienced single orgasms nevertheless reported a "physiological need" for multiple orgasms.

Penile-vaginal intercourse is only one of the many kinds of sexual activity that human couples engage in. Another is penile-anal intercourse. Anal intercourse is common (though by no means universal) among gay men. It is also surprisingly common in male-female sex: surveys indicate that at least 10% of American women, and much higher proportions in some other cultures, regularly engage in anal intercourse with their male partners. From the point of view of the insertive partner, anal intercourse differs in only minor respects from vaginal intercourse. But what about the receptive partner? Is the anus a sexual organ at all, or does the receptive partner participate merely to gratify his or her bedfellow, to avoid pregnancy, or for some purely psychological reason such as a Freudian "anal fixation"?

Although few men or women reach orgasm from anal stimulation alone, the anus is without question a sexual organ. For one thing, significant numbers of heterosexual women (about 10% of the respondents in one survey) use anal penetration, in conjunction with stimulation of the clitoris, during masturbation to orgasm—namely, in a situation where partner gratification and fear of pregnancy are irrelevant. Also, the perianal skin, the anal mucosa, and the anal sphincter are all richly innervated and capable of generating erotic sensation, and internal stimulation (for example, of the prostate gland in men) may also play an important role in the erotic significance of anal intercourse.

This is not to deny that the other factors mentioned above may contribute to the choice of anal intercourse over other sexual practices. For example, surveys report that women engage in anal intercourse more frequently with bisexual men than with exclusively heterosexual men—presumably because of a desire for anal intercourse on the part of their partners. The high incidence of heterosexual anal intercourse in some predominantly Catholic countries may partly result from fear of pregnancy combined with the unavailabity of contraceptive devices. Finally, some gay men have a strong life-long preference for receptive anal intercourse (see chapter 12). Some early researchers asserted that in these gay men the nerves that normally innervate the penis are misrouted to the anus. Today such claims seem ludicrous. It is much more probable that the pelvic anatomy of these men is the same as in other men, and that their preference for receptive anal intercourse reflects two factors: the sexual nature of the anus, which all individuals are capable of experiencing, combined with a psychological need for bodily penetration as a component of sex. This need may be shared by many women, but not by most heterosexual men or by gay men who take part in receptive anal sex on a more sporadic or opportunistic basis.

Although this is not a how-to book, I cannot mention the subject of anal sex without stressing that taking the receptive role in unprotected anal intercourse is the sexual practice that carries the highest risk of infection with the AIDS virus. Not only is it the riskiest type of gay sex, it is also believed to be considerably riskier than vaginal intercourse in male-female sex. Anyone who practices anal sex should use a condom.

Of course, there are many other types of sexual activity that humans (and animals) indulge in. Among lesbian women, for example, manual or oral stimulation of the clitoris is common. Mutual clitoral stimulation ("genito-genital rubbing") is seen among anthropoid apes, suggesting that the techniques of lesbian sexuality, like those of male-female and gay male sex, predate the evolution of the human species.

7

A Joy Proposed

Courtship Behavior

Animals—including humans—spend an inordinate amount of time getting ready to have sex. Something that could be achieved by mutual agreement in a minute or two is commonly drawn out into hours, days, even weeks of assiduous pursuit, comical misadventure, and brain-numbing stress. In a word: courtship.

The intricacies of courtship behavior take their origin in the imbalance of power that exists between the sexes. As outlined in chapter 2, females have taken upon themselves the greater share of the burden of producing and nurturing offspring. As a consequence, they have acquired the power to choose a mate from among a large number of more-or-less redundant males. Typically, they use this power either to select a male who exhibits qualities likely to favor the survival of their offspring, or to insist that the male invests in some fashion in the task of reproduction. Courtship is the demonstration of these qualities or the performance of this investment by the male, and the selection or rejection of the male by the female.

This is not to say that the female's role is simply that of a judge at a county fair, i.e., to view a parade of studs and to award her rosette to the winner. Although the male's role in courtship tends to be more active and demonstrative, the female often plays an active role too. In some species of songbird, for example, the female does not just listen to the male's courtship song but actually sings a duet with him. Female monkeys may actively solicit mounting by presenting their rump to the male, by flicking their tongues, or by staring at the male. Among rats a rapid wiggling of the ears is an especially effective come-on. Such behavior is termed *proceptive,* to distinguish it from *receptive* behavior where the female simply permits, or does not permit, copulation in response to the male's advances. Among humans, of course, women can take a very active part in courtship. Furthermore, the existence of physical attributes in women that are believed to have been influenced by sexual selection, such as relatively hairless bodies and large breasts, implies that partner choice by men as well as women plays a significant role in human mating. Most probably, the more symmetrical sex roles seen in human courtship are related to the more equal investment in child-rearing made by men and women, compared with the strongly female-biased investment seen in most other mammals.

Let us look at a couple of examples of courtship behavior in animals which throw some light on the biological mechanisms involved. A particularly interesting example is birdsong, which has been studied intensively by many brain scientists, but most especially by Fernando Nottebohm and his colleagues at the Rockefeller University.

Among most songbirds, only males sing, or males sing more frequent and elaborate songs than do females. Their song generally has at least two functions: maintaining a territory and attracting females. Males learn their songs early in life by listening to the songs of other birds. In some species a male bird's song repertoire, once learned, remains much the same throughout the bird's life. In others, such as the canary, new phrases are added to the song each year, and others are dropped. In addition, the phrases are combined in new ways to generate new songs.

The nuclei that are responsible for the generation of song are generally larger in the brains of male than female birds. This sexual dimorphism, like that in the rat's spinal cord described in the previous chapter, results from differences in hormone levels during early life: Mark Gurney, working at CalTech, administered masculinizing steroids to newly hatched female zebra finches and found that these birds developed song nuclei of a size typical for males. It is not known whether the steroids act directly on the neurons of the song nuclei, or indirectly as was the case with the rat spinal neurons.

A remarkable feature of the songbird's brain is that neurons are generated throughout life. In mammals, as will be discussed more fully in chapter 10, neurons are generated only during early development, before the neural circuits begin to function. In some of the vocal centers of songbirds' brains, however, Goldman and Nottebohm showed that new neurons are continuously being generated and inserted into preexisting, functioning circuits, while other neurons are dropping out. At first, it seemed as if the neurons that were being inserted or deleted might somehow encode the fragments of song that were being added or lost. But more recent findings indicate that this intriguingly simple notion is not an adequate description of what is going on. For one thing, new neurons are generated throughout the year, not just during the fall when songbirds are adding new phrases to their songs. Also, addition of new neurons occurs even in those species of songbirds that do not change their song from year to year. So, while the continuous replacement of neurons doubtless plays an important role in the production and modification of the bird's song, the precise nature of this role remains to be defined.

Another interesting feature of the circuitry responsible for birdsong is that it is often asymmetrical. In some species of birds, such as canaries, the left side of the brain generates the bulk of the song repertoire, while the right side contributes only a few syllables. In zebra finches, on the other hand, it is the right hemisphere that is primarily responsible for song production. There is a parallel here to the language system in humans, which also is a strongly lateralized function (it is generally located in the left hemisphere).

Unlike human language, birdsong is devoid of syntax or grammar; nor, indeed, is any meaning communicated by the detailed structure of the song, however elaborate it may be. To some extent, birdsong may represent useless labor forced on the male by the female, comparable to the building of bowers by male bowerbirds, as discussed in chapter 2. The male may in effect be saying "I'm such an efficient bird that I'm left with hours to waste on singing—so I would surely make an excellent husband."

The female, however, does have to listen to the song and process what she hears, at least to the extent of recognizing the species, and perhaps the local dialect or other finer characteristics of the song. In fact, female songbirds do have vocal systems in their brains, even in species where the females do not sing at all. The females may use their vocal systems to analyze the males' songs that they hear. If an adult female canary is treated with masculinizing hormones, she can be induced to begin singing, and there is a concomitant increase in the size of the vocal centers in her brain. This size increase seems to involve a hypertrophy of the preexisting neurons, and a formation of new synaptic connections, but not the generation of new neurons.

As a second example of courtship behavior let's take the phenomenon of eye contact. In primates, including humans, eye contact is a mutual behavior that is loaded with significance. It may represent a struggle for dominance between rivals, or, as anyone who has spent time in a singles bar or a gay bar will be aware, it can be a powerful cue to sexual arousal. Primates have developed uncannily precise mechanisms for determining, from the visual image of another individual's eyes, whether or not that individual is looking at them. Apparently this information, along with information about the other individual's facial expressions and behavior, is transmitted by a chain of synaptic connections from the visual regions of the cerebral cortex to the hypothalamus, where it influences the activity of neurons involved in the generation of sexual behavior. Conversely, the state of sexual arousal, represented in part at least by the activity of hypothalamic neurons, itself influences eye-contact behavior.

The role of eye contact in the courtship behavior of captive marmoset monkeys has been studied by Alan Dixson and S. A. C. Lloyd at the Centre for Reproductive Biology at Edinburgh, Scotland. In a typical encounter, the female marmoset would begin the sequence by freezing and staring at the male. If, and only if, the male returned eye contact and held it for a period of seconds, the female would proceed to the next stage, a bout of rapid tongue-flicking. The male would in turn flick his own tongue, and approach and attempt to mount the female. If she allowed him achieve the correct position on top of her, copulation and ejaculation would occur.

The completion of this series of events is contingent on a number of factors. First is the hormonal status of the female. She is more likely to stare at the male around the time of ovulation than at any other time in the estrous cycle. This is because of the high level of estrogens in the female's blood around the time of ovulation. Thus, if a female's ovaries (her source of estrogens) are removed surgically she spends much less time staring at the male, but the behavior recovers if she is given estrogens by injection. Second, the likelihood that the male will return the stare depends on his own internal state: he is less likely to do so if he is in the refractory period soon after ejaculating, or if his hypothalamus has been surgically lesioned.

Another more nebulous factor is the sexual attractiveness of the partner. The role of this factor is more obvious in situations where an animal (or human) has a choice among partners. Steven Pomerantz and his colleagues at the Wisconsin Regional Primate Research Center studied the sexual behavior of rhesus monkeys in "three-ways": one male in a cage with two estrous females. They found that the male directed nearly all his sexual advances to one of the two females, and she in turn would perform much more proceptive behavior than the other female. This exhibition of partner preference by the males was not caused by any absolute difference in attractiveness between the two females, however, since different males did not consistently prefer the same female. It is not known what brain circuits are responsible for this type of partner preference. They do, however, appear to be influenced by the blood levels of androgens during prenatal life: Pomerantz and colleagues reported that this type of partner preference is shown by male monkeys or by genetic females that were exposed to testosterone before birth, but not by females who were not given testosterone prenatally, even if their ovaries were removed at birth and they were treated with testosterone as adults.

Obviously, the details of courtship behavior differ radically from species to species. Yet in most species courtship behavior is influenced by the circulating levels of gonadal steroids, both in fetal life and in adulthood. It seems probable that these hormones influence courtship behavior in humans, although human courtship has strong cultural elements too. Even these cultural elements, however, can often be interpreted in terms of biological or sociobiological forces that act on many species. For example, the tradition of an engagement period lasting for several months before marriage, common in many human societies, could be interpreted as a mechanism to ensure that the woman does not come to the marriage already pregnant and hence fool the husband into rearing a child that is not his own. As we saw in chapter 2, even langur monkeys are capable of attempting such deception, so it is likely that evolution has favored the development by males of behavioral strategies to prevent such attempts from being successful.

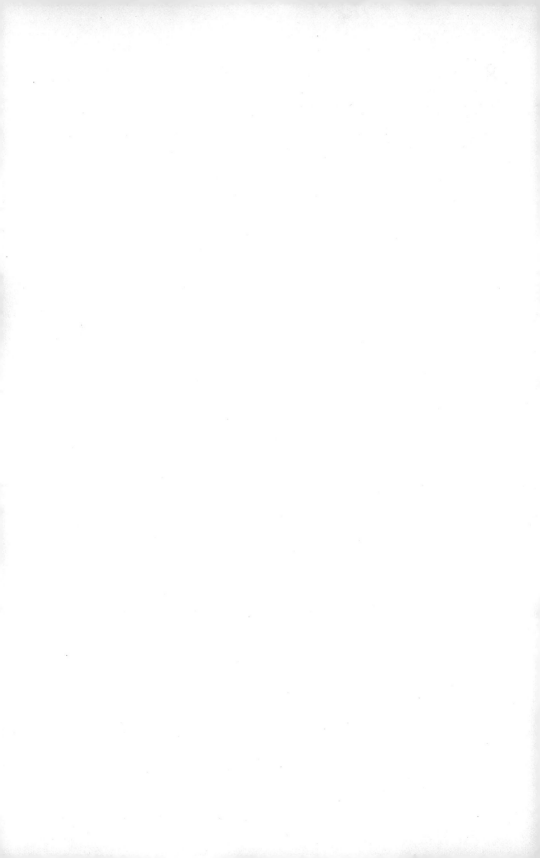

8

The Child-Changed Mother

Maternal Behavior

Why do parents, and especially mothers, devote so much time and effort to their children's welfare? The reason, in an evolutionary sense, was discussed in chapter 2: mothers have made such a large investment in their offspring by the time they are born that they are compelled to protect their investment by every means possible. But what is the mechanism by which this theoretical necessity is translated into action?

If one asks mothers themselves why they behave the way they do, they may rationalize their behavior in terms of self-interest by saying, "I do it so that I will have someone to look after me when I am old" or "I do it so as not to be arrested for child neglect," but more likely they will simply say "I do it because I love my child." To an outside observer, though, this love cannot be observed except in the mother's loving behavior, so that her statement translates into "I do it because I do it," or simply "I don't know why I do it." Any further understanding of the matter requires opening a mother's head and looking inside.

Whether rat mothers also love their offspring is hard to say, but they certainly act as if they do. Prior to giving birth, the female rat constructs a nest for her litter. Immediately after giving birth, she crouches over her pups to give them warmth and to allow them to suckle. She will retrieve pups that crawl away from the nest, and she licks her pups to clean them and to encourage them to empty their bladders (see chapter 10). She will also defend the pups aggressively against intruders. By contrast, if one gives a litter of newborn pups to a female rat who has not just given birth, she will not show any of these behaviors (although she will begin to do so gradually if given constant access to the pups for several days). What is different about the mother rat that causes her to show maternal behavior as soon as her pups are born?

The short answer is: hormones. In rats, the onset of maternity is accompanied by a reorganization of the brain under the influence of at least four hormones: estrogen, progesterone, prolactin, and oxytocin. The blood levels of the sex steroids estrogen and progesterone, produced by the ovaries, both increase during pregnancy, but shortly before the rat gives birth the level of progesterone declines to very low levels. This is a key signal for birth to occur, but in addition to triggering birth the fall in progesterone permits a corresponding rise in the levels of prolactin, a protein hormone secreted by cells in the pituitary gland under the influence of the hypothalamus. Prolactin is involved in preparing the mammary glands for the secretion of milk, but it also, in conjunction with estrogen, stimulates maternal behavior.

That hormones are indeed involved was demonstrated in striking experiments by Joseph Terkel and Jay Rosenblatt of Rutgers University. They surgically connected the bloodstreams of two rats, one a pregnant female about to give birth, and the other a female that was not pregnant and never had been pregnant. When the pregnant rat gave birth, she started acting maternally, but so did the second rat, under the influence of hormones entering her bloodstream from the mother rat.

Prolactin is the chief hormone involved, although it only exerts its effects when the rat has been primed by high levels of estrogens, such as are present toward the end of pregnancy. The importance of prolactin can be shown in the following way. The pituitary gland, source of prolactin and many other hormones, is surgically removed from a non-pregnant female rat. The rat is then treated with a sequence of estrogen and progesterone injections mimicking the hormonal changes occurring during pregnancy. At the time that would correspond to the birth of her offspring the rat is presented with a litter of newborn pups. Lacking her pituitary gland, she fails to show any maternal behavior, but she does so immediately if given an injection of purified prolactin.

Although prolactin itself is produced only by the pituitary gland, a group of hormones very similar to prolactin are produced by the placenta (or the placentas in the case of animals that carry multiple fetuses). These hormones, named *placental lactogens,* enter the mother's bloodstream in increasing amounts toward the end of pregnancy, and they may be even more important than the mother's own prolactin in stimulating maternal behavior immediately after the pups' birth. In a sense the fetus (or the fetoplacental unit) exerts mind control over its own mother by chemical means.

Prolactin and the placental lactogens act directly on the brain—specifically, on an anterior region of the hypothalamus that plays a role in the generation of maternal behavior. This has been shown (in mice) by injecting the hormones directly into this brain region: the injections elicit nest-building and pup retrieval. It is therefore likely that neurons in this region have receptors that bind prolactin, analogous to the steroid receptors that make some neurons sensitive to testosterone and other steroid hormones.

Oxytocin, as mentioned in chapter 5, is a small peptide hormone that is made by specialized neurons in the supraoptic and paraventricular nuclei of the hypothalamus. Their axons run down into the pituitary gland, where they release the hormone into the bloodstream. In addition, some oxytocin-containing neurons have axons that run to other parts of the brain and spinal cord, including the sexually dimorphic spinal nuclei that innervate the muscles of the penis. In males, as mentioned in chapter 6, oxytocin plays a role in orgasm. In females, a role in orgasm is uncertain, but three other functions are known. First, it is involved in giving birth (parturition): the hormone stimulates the contraction of the muscles of the uterus and thus helps expel the fetus. Second, it is involved in suckling: specifically, it causes ejection of milk from the ducts of the mammary glands into the nipples, where it can be obtained by the baby or pup. Third, it plays a role in generating maternal behavior.

The milk ejection reflex, and oxytocin's role in it, has been especially well studied. When a baby or pup sucks at the nipple, sensory fibers that innervate the nipple are activated, and they convey this information to the spinal cord, whence it is relayed over several synaptic links up the brain stem to the oxytocin-containing neurons in the supraoptic and paraventricular nuclei of the hypothalamus. The electrical activity of these neurons has been studied by microelectrode recording in female rats while they are nursing pups. During suckling, the oxytocin-containing neurons are put into an altered state in which, every few minutes, they give a short, rapid barrage of impulses (a "burst"). This burst occurs simultaneously among all the oxytocin neurons in both nuclei on both sides of the brain. The impulses are propagated down the axons of the neurons to their terminals in the pituitary gland. Here they cause release of oxytocin stored in the terminal enlargements of the axons, which are located close to blood vessels. The released hormone surges into the bloodstream and within a few seconds reaches the mammary glands, where it causes the muscles surrounding the mammary ducts to contract, expelling milk from the ducts into the nipples.

Most of the circuitry just described is present in female rats whether or not they have pups. In fact, it is present in male rats too. But there are specific changes in the supraoptic nucleus (and probably also in the paraventricular nucleus) toward the end of pregnancy that greatly facilitate the action of the milk ejection reflex. Barbara Modney and Glenn Hatton at Michigan State University examined the neurons in the supraoptic nucleus with electron microscopy. They found that in virgin rats each neuron is separated from its neighbors by very thin insulating layers produced by the non-neuronal supporting cells of the brain (the so-called *glial* cells). The same layers are present in pregnant rats. A few hours before the birth of the pups, however, these glial cell layers are withdrawn, and the oxytocin-containing neurons are allowed to come into direct contact with each other. Like the withdrawal of the graphite moderators in a nuclear reactor, this event allows the neurons to become much more excitable. The increased excitability may be due to the formation of specialized connections between neurons that permit the direct flow of electric current from one cell to another ("electrical coupling"). In addition, new synapses are formed in the supraoptic and paraventricular nuclei at about the same time, although the exact function of these synapses is not known. The structural changes are not permanent: toward the end of the period when the female is nursing her young the new synapses disappear and the glial layers again interpose themselves between adjacent neurons.

These findings illustrate that the brain is not a static object in adult life. Although, in mammals, no new neurons are added to the brain after the completion of development, new synaptic connections can be added, and other structural changes can occur that greatly affect the way neurons function. It may well be that synapses are broken and reformed by the millions in the regular course of daily life, but except in special circumstances such as those just described this anatomical remodeling is difficult to observe.

Some women describe episodes of intense pleasure akin to orgasm during nursing. It would be interesting to know whether the release of oxytocin during suckling plays a role in this subjective feeling, as it may do in actual orgasm.

Oxytocin also stimulates maternal behavior. As with prolactin, injection of oxytocin into the brain induces immediate maternal behavior in rats that have been primed with estrogens. Furthermore, drugs that block the effects of oxytocin (oxytocin antagonists) delay the appearance of maternal behavior in rats that have just delivered pups. Thus it appears that oxytocin does not act just on peripheral tissues such as the mammary glands and uterus, but also works within the brain. In fact, Thomas Insel of the National Institute of Mental Health, and other researchers, have shown that certain cell groups in the hypothalamus and nearby contain oxytocin receptors. The levels of these receptors are increased by exposure to high levels of estrogen, such as are seen toward the end of pregnancy. It is probable that the gene coding for the oxytocin receptor contains an estrogen response element—the short stretch of DNA which is recognized by the estrogen receptor—and that the binding of the estrogen receptor to this response element increases the rate at which the oxytocin receptor is synthesized.

Oxytocin has an interesting evolutionary history. It is almost identical to another peptide hormone, vasopressin, that is also synthesized by hypothalamic neurons and secreted from the pituitary gland. Vasopressin has a quite different role, being concerned primarily with the control of blood volume, yet eight of the nine amino acids that constitute the hormone are identical in the two peptides. In all vertebrates other than mammals there is only one such hormone, named vasotocin. This hormone differs by one amino acid from both vasopressin and oxytocin. It is likely that, early in the evolution of mammals, the vasotocin gene was duplicated, and that each of the two resulting genes, originally identical, mutated slightly to produce the oxytocin and vasopressin genes. The vasopressin gene remained primarily involved with the control of blood volume, while the oxytocin gene became involved in a set of functions—orgasm, giving birth, suckling, and maternal behavior—that are either unique to mammals or much better developed in mammals than in lower animals. From this point of view the duplication of the vasotocin gene—a genetic accident—was an important event in mammalian evolution.

So far, I have emphasized the controlling influence of hormones on maternal behavior. But hormones are by no means the whole story. In rats, only the maternal behavior displayed by the female immediately after delivery of the pups is dependent on hormones; any female rat, or juvenile rats of either sex, if given access to pups for a period of days, will gradually come to act maternally toward them. This gradual development of maternal behavior does not seem to be dependent on the hormones described above, and its basis is poorly understood.

The causes of maternal behavior in primates have been less extensively studied than in rodents. The general belief is that learning and social interactions play a more important role than do hormones. Juvenile monkeys have ample opportunity to witness maternal behavior directed toward themselves, their younger siblings, and other infants. Females will sometimes show maternal behavior to infants that are not their own. Such "aunting" behavior may have value as a rehearsal for true maternal behavior. Alternatively, it may be a form of altruism explicable by the theory of kin selection, as described in chapter 2. Either way, it must not depend on the hormonal changes accompanying pregnancy and birth, since the "aunts" are not necessarily mothers themselves.

Among primates, as among rats, maternal behavior is shown more frequently by females than males (indeed, that is why the behavior is called maternal). But male primates definitely have the capacity to show maternal behavior in some circumstances. For example, J. R. Gibber (of the University of Wisconsin) observed the responses of male and female rhesus monkeys to infant distress calls: when a male and female were tested together, the male sat back and acted as if the calls meant nothing to him, but when the male was tested alone he responded with alacrity. Similarly, it is not uncommon in the wild to observe male primates acting protectively toward infants when the mother or other females are unavailable.

It is clear then that sex differences in parental behavior, especially in primates, do not depend fully on prenatal organizational events in the brain. At the same time, there are hints that such prenatal events play some role, even in humans. As an example, John Money and Anke Ehrhardt (of Johns Hopkins University) reported that girls with congenital adrenal hyperplasia, who were exposed to abnormally high levels of androgens during late fetal life (see chapter 3), are significantly less interested in baby-sitting and other maternal-like behaviors than are other girls. The same appears to be true (although to a less marked extent) for girls who were exposed before birth to diethylstilbestrol (DES), according to a study by Ehrhardt and her colleagues. If these findings are correct, they would suggest that the levels of androgens usually present in male fetuses, while certainly not preventing the organization of circuits for maternal behavior, in some way restrict the range of circumstances in which such behavior is exhibited.

9

The Generation of Still-Breeding Thoughts

Brain Circuits for Sexuality

There are separate centers within the hypothalamus for the generation of male-typical and female-typical sexual behavior and feelings.

The foregoing, seemingly innocuous statement is calculated to raise the hackles of numerous critics. They will say: "How dare you define what is sex-typical behavior, thus branding anything else as pathological or deviant?" "How can you speak of a *center* for sex when we know that many brain regions are involved?" and "How can you say the hypothalamus has anything to do with *feelings* when feelings are conscious and must therefore be produced by the cerebral cortex and thalamus?"

While sticking to my guns, I do feel obliged to spell out what I mean by the above statement. First, I call behavior and feelings male-typical or female-typical when they are more common in one sex than the other. Taking the insertive role in sexual intercourse, for example, is male-typical behavior. Taking the receptive role is, for men, sex-atypical behavior. But in no way do I intend by this to label such behavior as undesirable or pathological.

Second, when I speak of a "center" for sex I mean that it is a crucial node in a complex circuit that involves many other brain regions. As stressed in chapter 4, the functions of a given brain nucleus are imbued in part by the incoming and outgoing connections it has with other parts of the brain. Removed and put in a dish, a "sex center" might give little hint that it was involved in sex rather than, say, walking or mathematics.

Finally, when I say a nucleus in the hypothalamus plays a role in the generation of sexual feelings I do not necessarily imply that these feelings reside in the hypothalamus. But I do imply that wherever these feelings reside, the hypothalamus plays a key role in triggering them.

Having fired off these defensive salvos, let me get on to the evidence for the existence of sexual centers in the hypothalamus. The evidence comes from ablation, stimulation, and recording experiments, and from studies of the chemistry and morphology of the regions involved.

Ablation studies (that is, studies involving the deliberate destruction of small regions of brain) have suggested that a region named the *medial preoptic area* plays a vital role in male-typical sexual behavior. This area lies toward the front of the hypothalamus, at or in front of the level of the optic chiasm (hence "preoptic") and close to the midline (hence "medial"). It is not a single nucleus but a region containing several small nuclei as well as axonal tracts. When this region is destroyed in male animals of many species, there is a reduction or complete cessation of the animal's heterosexual copulatory behavior—that is, the animal mounts females less readily or not at all. There is not a complete loss of sex drive, however. Monkeys whose medial preoptic areas have been damaged continue to masturbate (an activity that is commonly observed both in captive monkeys and in the wild). Male rats and ferrets that have received these lesions often show *increased* female-typical behavior (e.g., approach to a stud male, lordosis), especially when the operation is combined with estrogen treatment. The possible relevance of this observation to human homosexuality will be discussed in chapter 12.

Electrical stimulation of the medial preoptic area has the opposite effect. Of course, such experiments are rather crude because it is impossible to artificially generate the complex patterns of electrical activity that normally occur in a small brain region. Even so, the effects can be startling. A male monkey sitting idly with an estrous female (i.e., a female in heat) will, after a few seconds of stimulation, mount the female and commence pelvic thrusting. If the female is not in heat, however, the stimulation has little or no effect. It would appear, then, that the medial preoptic area does not simply generate a motor pattern of behavior (mounting) but rather generates an inner state in which appropriate signals from the female can readily elicit mounting.

Although stimulation of the medial preoptic area elicits mounting and pelvic thrusting, this artificially generated behavior does not usually culminate in ejaculation, at least in monkeys. For that, it appears that the activity of a closely adjacent cell group named the *dorsomedial nucleus* is required. Thus it seems that even within the general area of the anterior hypothalamus there is a parcellation of sexual functions among anatomically discrete regions.

Even more interesting evidence has come from experiments in which the natural electrical activity of single hypothalamic neurons is recorded while the animal is engaged in sexual behavior. Such experiments are particularly difficult to perform, because the animal's movements tend to dislodge the fine tip of the recording microelectrode from its desired location in immediate contact with the neuron being recorded. This difficulty was overcome in a rather artificial way by a research group at Kyushu University in Japan. The male monkey being studied was placed in a chair-like restraint and its head painlessly immobilized so that stable recordings could be made. The monkey was free to press a button, the effect of which was to bring toward him another chair in which sat an estrous female. When the two chairs were adjacent the two animals could copulate, albeit with some contortions, and without the male monkey moving its head. (The persistence of sexual behavior in these trying circumstances lends credence the old saying that "love will find a way").

In this study, the activity of many neurons in the medial preoptic area was found to be closely linked to the animal's state of sexual arousal. When the monkey caught sight of the female and pressed the button to bring her toward him, the cells discharged at a high rate (about 50 impulses per second). During copulation the discharge rate dropped, and after ejaculation it ceased almost completely, gradually recovering over a period of a half-hour or so as the monkey regained interest in the female. The specifically sexual nature of the neuronal activity was suggested by control experiments in which the other chair contained not a female monkey but a banana. In this case the monkey was equally avid in bringing the chair within reach, and he consumed the banana with enthusiasm, but the neuronal activity level was unaffected.

Putting all these observations together, it seems that the electrical activity of some neurons in the medial preoptic area may in some sense represent a male-typical sexual drive state. It is not certain where this information is sent to. Very possibly it is sent to several regions: to other hypothalamic regions such as the dorsomedial nucleus mentioned above, to lower centers in the brain stem where sexual reflexes such as penile erection are mediated, and (directly or indirectly) to the cerebral cortex, especially the motor regions that control the voluntary muscles involved in mounting and thrusting. But the detailed pattern of connections remains to be elucidated.

What is it that actually sets the activity level of the medial preoptic neurons? These neurons receive diverse inputs from numerous other brain regions. Among them are inputs from the olfactory system and from the cerebral cortex. In most animals (though less so in humans and other primates) smell is a key trigger for sexual activity. Rats, for example, use smell to distinguish the sex of another animal and indeed to recognize it as an individual. Even humans can readily tell the sex of another person by smell alone, and these olfactory cues may play a greater role in our sexual behavior than we commonly believe. Thus it is likely that sex-specific olfactory inputs can raise or lower the activity levels of hypothalamic neurons. The inputs from the cerebral cortex (many of which pass through a relay in a structure known as the *amygdala*) very likely mediate other sensory influences on sexual arousal. For example, some neurons in the monkey's visual cortex (and in the amygdala), discharge when the animal is viewing monkeys' faces. Some of these neurons only respond to the face of one particular individual monkey. It is reasonable to suspect that the activity of such neurons, transmitted to the medial preoptic area, might mediate the sexual arousal that certain faces induce in any particular individual. Of course, that's just speculation at this point. To pin it down further would require showing that just those neurons coding the faces of individuals that are attractive to the animal, or coding for the faces of a class of attractive individuals (e.g., females), have excitatory connections into the medial preoptic area.

Besides these neuronal inputs, the medial preoptic area also has major *hormonal* inputs. If a shot of radioactive testosterone is injected into an animal's bloodstream and the fate of the radioactivity is studied by autoradiography, it is found that medial preoptic neurons take it up at higher concentrations than any other brain region. The reason for this high uptake level is that these neurons have high levels of androgen receptors. This can be demonstrated by visualizing the receptors directly with immunocytochemistry, or by visualizing the activity of the androgen receptor gene with hybridization histochemistry (these techniques were described in chapter 5). In addition to androgen receptors, medial pre-optic neurons also have estrogen receptors, as well as the enzyme aromatase that converts androgens to estrogens.

A number of experiments have documented the important role sex steroids, and specifically testosterone, play in influencing the activity of medial preoptic neurons and hence in regulating male-typical sexual behavior. Removal of circulating androgens by castration, or blocking their effects with a specific antagonist, reduces the responsiveness of medial preoptic neurons and also reduces male-typical sex drive. This reduction takes several days or weeks, even in rats, and in humans it may take much longer. If a rat is castrated and as a consequence no longer mounts females, mounting behavior can be restored by directly applying minute amounts of testosterone to the medial preoptic area.

In rats, many of the effects of testosterone on the brain require conversion of the testosterone to estrogen. The main evidence for this is that testosterone-like drugs that activate androgen receptors but that cannot be converted to estrogen lack many of the behavioral effects of testosterone itself. In primates, on the other hand, it appears that many of testosterone's effects do not require this conversion.

As described in chapter 3, the effects of steroid hormones are primarily on gene expression. Testosterone does not directly excite or inhibit a neuron in the way that neurotransmitters do. There is, however, evidence that the genes whose expression is influenced by androgens and estrogens include several that code for enzymes or receptors involved in neuro-transmission. Thus the hormones are able to modulate the degree to which a neuron responds to an incoming input, such as a potentially exciting olfactory signal. It also seems probable that there are effects of testosterone on the formation or loss of synaptic connections, or on other cellular growth processes that affect function.

The medial preoptic region is sexually dimorphic: it contains at least one nucleus that is larger, on average, in males than females. This observation was first made in rats (by Roger Gorski and his colleagues at UCLA) and has since been confirmed in other rodents, as well as in the ferret (a carnivore) and in humans. The discovery of this anatomical dimorphism has been an important element in the elucidation of the mechanisms by which the sexual differentiation of the brain comes about.

The identification of the sexually dimorphic nucleus or nuclei in humans involved what seems to have been a false lead. In 1985, Dutch scientists reported the existence of a nucleus in the anterior hypothalamus which they claimed to be larger in men than in women. They termed this nucleus the *sexually dimorphic nucleus of the preoptic area (SDN-POA)*. This designation turned out to be unfortunate. First, the nucleus had already been given a name (the *nucleus intermedius*) by other researchers, and etiquette among neuroanatomists (as in so many other fields of exploration) demands that the first discoverer has the right to name whatever he or she discovers. Second, the nucleus did not correspond in position or appearance to the sexually dimorphic nucleus in the rat: instead of lying far medially, close to the third ventricle, it was positioned near the lateral margin of the region. Third, subsequent researchers (including myself) have failed to confirm any difference in the size of this nucleus in men and women.

More recently Gorski and his colleagues (in particular, his student Laura Allen) have reported that two other nuclei in the human preoptic area are larger in men than women. They named these two nuclei the second and third interstitial nuclei of the anterior hypothalamus (INAH 2 and INAH 3). (INAH 1, which they found not to be dimorphic, corresponded to the nucleus intermedius.) While the dimorphism in INAH 2 was somewhat equivocal and possibly limited to certain age groups, the dimorphism in INAH 3 was sizeable (about a threefold difference in volume between the sexes) and apparently independent of age. (Nevertheless, as I describe in chapter 12, there are size differences even within one sex that are at least partly associated with differences in sexual orientation.) Furthermore, the position and general appearance of INAH 3 corresponded quite well with the SDN of the rat. That is not to say that the structures in the two species are necessarily homologous: one would need to know more about their connections, chemical makeup, and soon, to be sure on that point.

We have seen two potential reasons why males show more male-typical sexual behavior than do females: first, the function of the medial preoptic area is influenced by androgens, which are present at much higher levels in the blood of males than of females. Second, at least one nucleus in the medial preoptic area is larger, on average, in males than in females. It is unlikely, however, that these two factors alone account for the sex differences in male-typical behavior. For one thing, raising the testosterone levels of adult females does not cause them to show the complete patterns of male-typical sexual behavior. (In women, administration of testosterone can increase sexual drive, but it does not change the nature of that drive.) Also, and somewhat surprisingly, lesions that destroy the sexually dimorphic nucleus in rats, but that spare the surrounding, nondimorphic parts of the medial preoptic area, actually seem to have little effect on the rats' sexual behavior.

It therefore seems likely that there are further, more subtle sex differences in the medial preoptic area that go beyond the simple matter of the size of the sexually dimorphic nucleus. In fact, at least two such differences are known. First, electron microscopic studies of the area have revealed differences between male and female rats in the shape and position of synapses made between neurons, and second, immunohistochemistry has shown sex differences in the distribution of several neurotransmitters in the region.

If the medial preoptic area is the principal hypothalamic region for male-typical sexual behavior, the corresponding region for female-typical sexual behavior lies a few millimeters further back, in a structure called the *ventromedial nucleus*. This nucleus lies at the level of the median eminence, close to the midline, and near the undersurface of the brain ("ventral"). It is a relatively large nucleus as hypothalamic nuclei go (it is about 3 mm across), and its functions are not exclusively sexual. For example, it is also involved in the regulation of feeding behavior: lesions in this nucleus can cause obesity. Most probably, the various functions of the ventromedial nucleus are carried out by anatomically distinct subregions, and in fact it appears to be the ventrolateral portion of the nucleus that is specifically involved with sex.

The evidence implicating the ventromedial nucleus in the regulation of female-typical sexual behavior comes from the same kind of experiment as just described for the medial preoptic area. Damage to the nucleus impairs or prevents female rats and monkeys from exhibiting their typical behavior (ear-wiggling, darting, and lordosis in rats, "presenting" in monkeys). Electrical stimulation of the nucleus elicits or facilitates this behavior. Recording experiments have shown that the activity of some neurons in the ventromedial nucleus is strongly correlated with receptive behavior, including copulation itself.

The ventromedial nucleus is also strongly influenced by sex steroids. In the female rat, whose sexual receptivity waxes and wanes dramatically with the estrous cycle, the major hormones involved are the ovarian hormones: estrogen and progesterone. The two hormones cooperate in an interesting way in eliciting receptive behavior. Estrogen works slowly, gradually priming the nucleus over a period of about 24 hours. Once primed, the nucleus can be activated by progesterone (applied via the circulation or directly injected into the nucleus) within an hour. The priming process seems to involve at least two major phenomena. First, during the 24 hours of exposure to estrogen, there are growth processes within the nucleus that include formation of new synaptic connections. Second, one of the effects of estrogen is to cause the neurons of the ventromedial nucleus to synthesize progesterone receptors. In technical parlance, the estrogen exposure "induces the expression" of progesterone receptors. This is why, in the absence of prior estrogen exposure, progesterone does not elicit female-typical behavior: the neurons simply do not have enough receptors for it to have a significant effect on them.

In rats, this key process, the induction of progesterone receptors in the ventromedial nucleus by estrogen, is sex-specific: it does not occur in adult male rats even if they are castrated before being given estrogen. Thus, progesterone does not facilitate the lordosis reflex in males, whether they are estrogen primed or not. This sex difference in the brain has its origin in events that occur prior to birth.

In female primates, including women, the behavioral effects of sex steroids are more subtle and complex. Removal of the ovaries (and hence of the main source of estrogen and progesterone) does not markedly reduce women's sex drive. Curiously, a more marked reduction in sex drive occurs in women (and female monkeys) after removal of the adrenal glands. These glands secrete measurable amounts of androgens, and it seems to be the loss of these androgens that is responsible for the reduction in sex drive, since administration of testosterone restores it to normal levels.

Why then do female monkeys show such great changes in sexual behavior around the estrous cycle? There is some evidence that it involves olfactory communication between the female and the male. When estrogen levels are high (prior to ovulation) odors arising from the vagina have a stimulatory effect on the male's mounting behavior; when estrogen levels are low and progesterone levels are high (after ovulation), the vaginal secretions have a different odor, which actually seems to discourage the male from mounting. Thus, if the perineal (sexual) skin of a female who is not in heat is coated with secretions taken from the vagina of a female who *is* in heat, the male will mount her. That these effects are truly mediated by olfactory cues is shown by experiments in which a male's olfactory sense is temporarily knocked out: such a male does not discriminate between females who are in heat and females who are not. The odorants are believed to be fatty acids produced by bacterial degradation of organic material in the estrogen-primed vagina. There is some suggestive evidence that a similar mechanism may operate in humans: men appear to initiate sex with women more often during the preovulatory phase of the menstrual cycle than during the postovulatory phase. Whether the men's behavior is regulated by olfactory cues remains to be studied.

It would make a pleasing symmetry if there were a sex dimorphism in the ventromedial nucleus opposite to that seen in the medial preoptic area; that is, if the nucleus were bigger in females than in males. That appears not to be the case, however. In fact, in rats the nucleus is slightly bigger in males than females. Why then do females show more female-typical sexual behavior that males? In rats, different hormone levels play a partial role, but that is not likely to be a major factor in primates. It is more likely that prenatal events lead to sex-distinct patterns of synaptic connections in the ventromedial nucleus. Another possibility is that the medial preoptic area exerts an inhibitory influence on the ventromedial nucleus; according to this idea, females exhibit more female-typical behavior than males because their ventromedial nucleus is subject to less inhibition from the medial preoptic area.

Perhaps the key unresolved issue with respect to the hypothalamus and sexual function is this: what is the *level* of control exerted by the hypothalamus? At one extreme one might think of it simply as a low-level center mediating simple behavioral acts such as mounting and lordosis. According to this idea, sexual motivation, state of arousal, sexual orientation, partner choice, and so forth are all generated elsewhere, perhaps in the cerebral cortex or amygdala: signals about these states must flow through the hypothalamus to actually become manifest in behavior. At the other extreme is the notion that the nuclei of the hypothalamus constitute high-level control centers that actually dictate sexual feelings regardless of whether any sexual behavior takes place.

Much of the animal research tends to reinforce the first view. But this may be misleading. We cannot readily ask animals about their inner states; it is much easier to simply observe their behavior and, for example, to note how this behavior is affected by damage to various hypothalamic structures. Simple behaviors such as mounting and lordosis are the easiest to observe and measure; thus there is a natural tendency to emphasize the role of the hypothalamus in generating these behaviors. Also, the very small size of many hypothalamic nuclei suggests to many people that they cannot be doing anything terribly complicated or high-level, such as might be implied by "feelings," "orientation," and so on.

Yet observations on humans who have had hypothalamic nuclei destroyed surgically tell quite a different story. Such operations were done (in West Germany in the 1960s) on men whose sexual behavior was considered pathological or sociopathic. Typically, the medial preoptic area and the ventromedial nucleus was destroyed. If the hypothalamus were a low-level center concerned only with the mechanics of sex, one might expect such men to say that they continued to desire and seek sexual partners, but that once in bed they couldn't perform. In fact, however, what many of these men reported was an overall reduction or loss of sexual feelings, desires, imagery, and drive, as well as of actual sexual behavior. This implies that an intact hypothalamus is required for the generation of sexuality in the broadest sense. Similarly, androgen-blocking drugs, which are sometimes given to sex offenders, tend to reduce their sexual thoughts and drive, not just their copulatory behavior. Since the hypothalamus is so rich in androgen receptors, one has to suspect that it is the drugs' action on this part of the brain that is responsible for the reduction in sexuality. (This is not so clean an experiment as the surgery, of course, because there are other brain regions, such as the amygdala, that also have high levels of androgen receptors.)

In trying to resolve this issue it is important to bear in mind that the connections between the hypothalamus and the rest of the brain, especially the cerebral cortex, are two-way; the cortex can influence the hypothalamus and the hypothalamus can influence the cortex. Unquestionably, sexual ideation and complex sexual behaviors such as choosing and seeking partners requires the activity of large regions of the cerebral cortex. One may assume that these regions send signals to the hypothalamus that, combined with olfactory inputs, sensory inputs from the genitalia, and sex hormones circulating in the bloodstream, set the level of activity of neurons in the medial preoptic area and ventromedial nucleus. These neurons in turn send signals down to the brain stem and spinal cord to influence the mechanics of sex, but they also send signals back to wide areas of the cerebral cortex that very likely influence sexual ideation and complex sexual behavior. Thus one can think of a cortex-hypothalamus-cortex circuit (actually it probably includes other structures such as the amygdala) whose activity as a whole is the key to sexual life. The medial preoptic area and the ventromedial nucleus may well be the prime nodes in this circuit: the nodes whose activity most purely represents the general level of sexual arousal. One might go beyond that to speculate that the activity levels of some neurons in the medial preoptic area represent male-typical arousal, while that of some neurons in the ventromedial nucleus represent female-typical arousal. This is a tempting notion, but one that goes well beyond the evidence presently available.

10

My Brain I'll Prove the Female

Sex and Brain Development

In the preceding chapter I described what we know of the mechanisms by which the hypothalamus generates male- and female-typical sexual behavior. There were some hints as to why sexual behavior differs between the sexes: the different levels of circulating sex hormones, the existence of a sexually dimorphic nucleus in the medial preoptic area, and the differences in synaptic architecture and neurotransmitters. To better appreciate the reasons for differences between the sexes, however, we need to ask how this part of the brain develops in a sex-differentiated fashion.

The brain and spinal cord start out as a simple hollow tube running the length of the body. The fluid-filled space inside the tube eventually becomes the system of *ventricles* within the brain. The cells forming the inner lining of the tube divide repeatedly, and their daughter cells migrate outward from this inner lining to form the nuclear and cortical structures of the mature nervous system. At the level of the spinal cord this growth process is relatively modest, so that the original tube-like structure is preserved. At the level of the brain, however, cell division continues much longer, and the masses of daughter cells, migrating in various and sundry directions, cause the walls of the tube to swell and buckle into a highly contorted shape. As the neurons tire of their youthful wanderings and settle down into a sedentary adulthood, they establish the *gray matter* of the brain, and they put out processes (*axons*) that form synaptic connections with other cells. Huge bundles of axons running from one part of the brain to another form the *white matter;* these axonal tracts further confuse the original tubular pattern.

The neurons of the hypothalamus originate by division of cells lining the portion of the tube that becomes the *third ventricle,* the midline cleft that separates the left and right halves of the hypothalamus. Thus they only have to migrate a short distance sideways to take up their final positions in the various hypothalamic nuclei.

An ingenious technique allows one to permanently label particular sets of developing neurons and to subsequently follow their development and ultimate fate. During the initial period of repeated cell division (mitosis), each cell must transcribe all its chromosomes prior to each division in order to provide a full set for each of its two daughters. This requires the incorporation of the four chemicals in which the genetic code is written (A,G,C, and T) into new strands of DNA. If, during the time when a particular cell is doubling its chromosomes, the animal is administered a radioactive version of one of these chemicals (usually T or thymidine), the radioactivity itself is incorporated into the DNA of the daughter cells. If the daughter cells continue to divide, the radioactivity is diluted out with each subsequent division and eventually becomes undetectable, but if the daughter cells cease to divide and begin their migration, the radioactivity remains at the same high level for as long as the cells live, which is often for the entire life of the animal. (There will be some decline due to the gradual decay of the radioactivity itself, but if a long-lived isotope such as tritium [^{3}H] or carbon 14 is used this will not be a major problem.) The presence of the radioactivity can be detected at any time by killing the animal, slicing the brain, and performing autoradiography. As described in chapter 5, this technique causes the radioactively labeled cells to become overlaid with silver grains that can be seen and counted under the microscope.

This technique has been used by Gorski and his colleagues to study the development of the sexually dimorphic nucleus (SDN) in the medial preoptic area in rats. They found that administration of ^{3}H-thymidine to rat fetuses on the eighteenth day of gestation (i.e., about 5 days before birth) permanently labeled many neurons in the SDN, indicating that these neurons went through their last division on that day. About the same number of cells became labeled in males and females, but during a short period around and just after birth many of the labeled cells in female pups died, leaving a nucleus that contained more cells in males than in females.

Why did the neurons in the female pups die? I discussed this question earlier with respect to the sexually dimorphic nucleus in the rat's spinal cord (chapter 6). In that case the evidence indicated that the death of motor neurons in the spinal cord of the female rat pups was secondary to the loss of muscles in the developing female genitalia: the neurons died because they had nothing to innervate. The loss of the target muscles was itself due to a lack of sufficient levels of circulating androgens to keep the muscles alive.

What about the neurons of the sexually dimorphic nucleus? These neurons do not innervate muscles but instead make synaptic connections with other neurons in the brain. Here too, however, the levels of androgens in the blood are crucial. If a male pup's own source of testosterone (its testes) is removed, or if it is given a drug that prevents testosterone from binding to its receptors in the brain, the numbers of labeled cells in the nucleus will decline as they do in females. Conversely, if a female pup is given testosterone in amounts mimicking those normally present in male pups, the number of labeled cells will remain at the high levels typical of males. So it is the level of circulating testosterone during a *critical period,* extending from about 3 days prior to birth until about 6 days after birth, that determines the size of the sexually dimorphic nucleus and the number of neurons within it. As with the vocal nuclei in the brains of songbirds (see chapter 7), it is not certain whether testosterone acts directly on the neurons of the nucleus to promote their survival, or whether the effect is indirect. Since these neurons possess high levels of androgen receptors, however, a direct effect is a good possibility. Furthermore, an effect on the neurons themsleves is suggested by the observation that injection of minute quantities of testosterone directly into the anterior hypothalamus of female rat pups can partially prevent the normal cell death.

The effect of testosterone on the development of the SDN is called *organizational* because it permanently influences the organization of the brain in a way that affects behavior much later in life. There are probably a large number of such organizational effects of testosterone, most of them less visually striking than its effect on the size of the SDN, but still of major functional significance. These other effects include the development of sex-specific patterns of synaptic connectivity, and sex-specific expression of genes, neurotransmitters, and so on. They involve not just the hypothalamus but also many other parts of the brain—androgen receptors are widespread in the brain during prenatal life. As is true of the rest of the body, the brain's intrinsic developmental program is female; as far as we know this program does not require any hormonal or other intructions. It takes a specific external signal, the presence of sufficient circulating levels of androgens, to reprogram development in the male direction. These organizational effects stand in contrast to the effects of gonadal steroids in adulthood, which are termed activational: their effects are to bring preexisting circuits into operation and to keep them in operation for as long as the steroid is present.

The organizational effects of testosterone have major consequences for the animal's behavior. Even before puberty, the behavior of male and female animals differs. In monkeys, for example, male young participate in more rough-and-tumble play than do females. This discrepancy results from the difference in androgen levels during prenatal life: as shown by Robert Goy and colleagues at the University of Wisconsin, females exposed to raised levels of testosterone prenatally show increased rough-and-tumble play, while males whose testosterone levels were lowered prenatally show less rough-and-tumble play. There is evidence for similar effects in humans. Sheri Berenbaum (of Chicago Medical School) and Melissa Hines (of UCLA) tested the toy preference of young (2- to 4-year-old) children. They found that most boys had a preference for toys like model trucks over dolls, while girls tended to play with trucks and dolls about equally. Girls who had been exposed to unusually high levels of androgens prenatally, as a result of congenital adrenal hyperplasia (see chapter 3), showed the toy preference typical of boys. It seems likely therefore that the sex differences in the play behavior of children, both in terms of toy preference and rough-and-tumble play, are influenced by the organizational effects of high or low levels of prenatal androgens. This is not to rule out an effect of parental influence, but this influence may be less significant than is commonly believed.

Some play behavior among both animals and humans has strong sexual content. Play-mounting is common among young monkeys of both sexes; with increasing age (but still before sexual maturity) male monkeys adopt a style of mounting called the "double foot-clasp mount" in which they support themselves on their partner's hind legs rather than on the ground. This behavior, very similar to that shown by mature males during actual copulation, is strongly dependent on androgen exposure during fetal life, as may readily be shown by administering androgens or androgen blockers appropriately. As for humans, it is very possible that children's roles in "Playing Doctor," "Seven Minutes in Heaven," and other sexual games of which parents generally seem so blissfully unaware, are also under the organizational influence of prenatal androgens, although there is no direct evidence to support this idea.

The level of androgens during development has an even more dramatic effect on sexual behavior in adulthood. If male rat pups are castrated at or prior to birth and allowed to grow up, they fail to show male-typical sexual behavior, even if they are given testosterone. Furthermore, if these rats, as adults, are given estrogen and progesterone, mimicking the hormonal milieu of adult female rats, they will display lordosis when paired with a stud male. But if the castration is not performed until a few days *after* birth, neither of these effects occur: as adults testosterone induces male-typical behavior and estrogen plus progesterone fails to induce female-typical behavior. So the sex-typical behavior is organized during the critical period around the time of birth, even though the behavior itself is not seen till much later. The situation with female pups is similar: giving testosterone during the critical period allows them, as adults, to show male-typical behavior and prevents them from showing female-typical behavior.

Another important organizational effect of androgens in rats has to do with the estrous cycle. During the female rat's cycle, the rise in circulating estrogen (derived from the maturing ovarian follicle) in the first part of the cycle is followed by a surge in the secretion of *luteinizing hormone* from the pituitary gland. Luteinizing hormone is required for the final maturation of the developing oocyte: without it, the follicle and the oocyte it contains will die. This surge in luteinizing hormone secretion in response to high estrogen levels in the blood occurs only in female rats, and not in males, even when males are given large doses of estrogen. But female rats that, as young pups, were given a single dose of testosterone will fail to show the luteinizing hormone surge as adults, and in fact will not cycle or ovulate at all. Similarly, male pups castrated at birth *will* show a luteinizing hormone surge in response to estrogen when they are adults. The critical period for the organization of the luteinizing hormone response appears to extend from birth until about the tenth day of life; this is slightly later than the critical period for the organization of the morphological sex differences in the sexually dimorphic nucleus.

The manner in which estrogen triggers the luteinizing hormone surge is complex and not fully understood. Luteinizing hormone is secreted from specialized glandular cells in the pituitary gland. The release of the hormone is controlled primarily by another hormone, appropriately named *luteinizing hormone–releasing hormone* (LHRH). This is one of the hormones, briefly mentioned in chapter 5, that is secreted by neurons in the hypothalamus and then conveyed by special blood vessels along the stalk that connects the brain to the pituitary gland. Once in the pituitary gland, LHRH stimulates release of luteinizing hormone into the general circulation. The neurons in the hypothalamus that synthesize and secrete LHRH seem not to be directly influenced by estrogen; rather they are under the control of yet another set of neurons, situated in a tiny nucleus at the very front of the hypothalamus whose name is altogether too long and cumbersome to burden you with. Its abbreviation is AVPV. AVPV is slightly bigger in female than in male rats, and contains more cells that use certain neurotransmitters, such as dopamine. Many neurons in AVPV carry receptors for estrogen and progesterone. Damage to this nucleus in female rats prevents the luteinizing hormone surge. Thus there is a cascade of events (probably even more complex than sketched here) that leads from the raised blood level of estrogen to the surge of luteinizing hormone. The need for such a complex chain of events is unclear, although presumably its function is to allow for modification or fine-tuning of the hormonal response by other hormonal or neuronal processes.

It is not known for sure which part of this cascade is organized in a sex-differentiated fashion during the critical period, nor what the process of organization consists of. But the AVPV is a good candidate to be the site, because of the morphological and neurochemical sex differences that exist there, and because this nucleus (like the sexually dimorphic nucleus in the medial preoptic area) is very rich in androgen receptors. It is interesting that testosterone seems to have opposite effects in the two nuclei during the critical period: promoting development in the SDN and slowing it in the AVPV. Presumably the genes that are controlled by androgen receptors are different in the two nuclei.

One reason for mentioning the luteinizing hormone surge and its development is that according to some scientists the presence or absence of this surge in humans distinguishes between homosexual and hetero-sexual individuals. As we shall see later, however (chapter 12), this claim seems to depend upon a false assumption about the equivalence of hormonal mechanisms in rats and humans.

So far, I have rather implied that there are only two normal avenues of development, a male-typical avenue, taken by males, and a female-typical avenue, taken by females. I have described diversions from these avenues only in the context of clearly abnormal events such as castration or the administration of synthetic hormones. It is important to under-stand, however, that there is considerable variability in sexual behavior even among animals of the same sex, and that to some extent this variability can be traced to processes that occur naturally during devel-opment.

Female rats vary in the frequency of lordosis and in circumstances in which it can be elicited. In addition, it is not uncommon for female rats to mount other receptive females, to perform pelvic thrusting and even to show the motor patterns that accompany ejaculation. Lynwood Clemens (of Michigan State University) discovered that the readiness of a female rat to display this male-typical sexual behavior is greatly influenced by its position in the uterus when it was a fetus. Rats, of course, carry several fetuses at the same time, and these fetuses are lined up within the two tubular horns of the uterus like oranges stuffed into a pair of socks. Clemens found that female fetuses that happen to lie between male fetuses are more likely to display mounting behavior as adults than are fetuses that lie between female fetuses. More recently it has been shown that the crucial factor is the presence of a male fetus on the side of the female between her and the cervix. This is the "upstream" side, in the sense that the flow of blood along the uterine vessels is from the cervix toward the ovary. It seems likely, therefore, that a chemical signal travels in the bloodstream from the male to the female fetus and influences her later sexual behavior. In all probability this signal is tes-tosterone itself, produced in the gonads of the male fetus. In fact, female fetuses situated in contiguity to males do have higher blood levels of testosterone than those situated between females, and at birth their external genitalia are partially masculinized—evidence of testosterone exposure.

It is unclear whether the uterine contiguity effect has any functional significance. Is it merely an undesired side-effect of the female rat's reproductive physiology, or is it advantageous (in a sociobiological sense) for a female rat to produce female offspring who are behaviorally diverse? One cannot answer this question with any certainty. It is interesting, however, that females exposed to androgens by the contiguity effect are partially masculinized not only in their sexual behavior, but also in some other behaviors including aggressiveness and exploratory behavior. These behaviors are very important in terms of survival value, and any estimation of the value of the uterine contiguity effect would have to take all these traits into account.

Of course, the contiguity effect has little direct relevance to human sexuality, since most human fetuses are singletons. Even in the case of twins, it is unlikely that a male fetus could significantly masculinize his female co-twin, because the blood supplies of human twin fetuses are more independent of each other than is the case with rat fetuses. Nevertheless, it points up the possibility that it might be advantageous to produce, by one means or another, offspring displaying some diversity in sexual behavior.

Diversity in sexual behavior is found among male rats too. If a number of normal, off-the-shelf male rats are paired with receptive females, some of the males are much more sexually active than others. Richard Anderson and his colleagues at Brigham Young University showed that the rats that are more active have, on average, a larger sexually dimorphic nucleus than the less active rats. Thus, even among normal male rats there is a correlation between the size of the nucleus and male-typical sexual behavior. Whether the rats with the smaller nuclei could be more readily induced to display female-typical behavior such as lordosis was not tested.

One factor that very clearly influences the sexual behavior of male rats is stress. Not stress on the male rats themselves as adults, but stress on their mother when they were fetuses. This "maternal stress effect" was discovered by Ingeborg Ward at Villanova University. The stress does not have to be very extreme or prolonged. A typical regimen involves confinement of the pregnant female rat in a Plexiglas tube under bright lights. This treatment is given for 45 minutes, three times a day, for the last week of pregnancy. When the sexual behavior of the male offspring of this pregnancy is tested, they are found to display mounting behavior less readily, and lordosis behavior more readily, than the male offspring of females who were not stressed.

The reason for this effect of maternal stress is probably that it alters the levels of testosterone in the developing fetus. In unstressed fetuses, testosterone levels reach a peak around the eighteenth and nineteenth days of development, just at the onset of the critical period for the development of the sexually dimorphic nucleus in the medial preoptic area. In stressed fetuses, the testosterone peak occurs earlier, around the sixteenth and seventeenth day, and by the eighteenth day the level of the hormone has fallen to below that seen in unstressed fetuses. These levels are insufficient for the survival and growth of the complete set of SDN neurons, and generally the nucleus ends up intermediate in size between the typical male and the typical female nucleus. Other organizational processes are very likely also affected by the lower testosterone levels.

Unlike the uterine contiguity effect, the maternal stress effect is potentially relevant to human sexual development, since many women are exposed to stress during pregnancy. This topic will be taken up again in the context of sexual orientation (chapter 12).

These two effects (uterine contiguity and maternal stress) are environmental, in the sense that they are effects exerted on the individual from outside the individual itself, but they are prenatal. What about such effects after birth, when the individual is in direct contact with the world and all its vicissitudes?

For every newborn mammal, the piece of the environment that looms largest is its mother. It is universally acknowledged that the manner in which a mother treats her offspring plays an important role in the offspring's psychological development, including the development of its sexuality. What is perhaps less well understood is that the infant itself exerts considerable control over its mother's behavior.

A particularly well-studied example is the habit of mother rats of licking the anogenital region of their offspring. By doing this the mother stimulates urination by the offspring, and she also imbibes most of the urine produced. This behavior will doubtless strike many readers as uncouth, perhaps confirming their image of rats as unlovely pests whose lives should in no way be taken as models for our own. In extenuation I should point out, first, that this behavior is an exemplary case of recycling what for rats is a precious resource—water. Second, unattractive animals do not have a monopoly on unattractive behavior: one has only to think of that adorable creature, the mother koala bear, and her habit of feeding her offspring with her own feces. Finally, whether or not the lives of rats resemble our own, they do have two major advantages as research subjects: they are cheap and they grow up quickly. In today's world of tight budgets and short attention spans, these advantages outweigh any possible shortcomings.

As I was saying, mother rats lick their male and female pups differently. Specifically, they lick the anogenital regions of male pups more than female pups. Rats tell the sex of their offspring by smell, and if the mother is prevented from smelling her offspring (by destruction of her olfactory mucosa), all offspring will be licked at the lower rates normal for female pups. The male pups who are exposed to this (for males) abnormally low rate of licking will later show differences in their sexual behavior: they will mount females less readily and take longer to reach ejaculation than rats that, as pups, were licked at the higher rate. It is likely that the effect of the high rate of licking is to increase the production of testosterone by the male pup's testes, but how this comes about is unclear.

On the face of it this is a bizarre chain of events. Male rat pups know what sex they are (or rather they act as if they know, since they put out the appropriate male-specific odor for their mother to recognize), so why should they require this "validation" of their maleness from their mothers to achieve normal male-typical sexual behavior as adults? Why not skip this loop through the environment and rely simply on an internally directed developmental program that progresses to male-typical behavior regardless of what the mother does or does not do to her young? There is no clear answer to this question, but, as with most complex control systems in biology, the reason probably has to do with the possibility for fine-tuning that the extra steps offer. Much information is available to the mother that is not available to the pups: information about food availability, population density, and so on, that might well affect the reproductive strategy that is likely to be most appropriate for her young. It may be that her licking behavior in essence communicates some of this information to the pups. Indeed, it is possible that the maternal stress effect, discussed above, should be viewed in the same light: stressors such as crowding and malnutrition could well be signals that indicate a need for an altered reproductive strategy. But proving the functional significance of these effects would require more complex and lengthy experiments than have so far been undertaken.

Human mothers also treat male and female infants differently. It has been reported that they spend more time holding males than females, for example. How male infants persuade their mothers to do this is uncertain: maybe they simply cry more. There is no evidence that this differential treatment has any long-term effects on the children's sexual development. Nevertheless there are many examples of human parental behavior that *have* been claimed to influence the offspring's sexuality. In classic psychoanalytic theory, for example, parental behavior was held to be a key factor in the determination of an individual's sexual orientation. This notion is discussed further in chapter 12.

During the period between weaning and puberty—the period that is so remarkably long in humans—the interactions between an individual and other juveniles contribute to the individual's developing sexuality. Robert Goy and his colleagues have made a detailed study of the effects of rearing young male rhesus monkeys in isolation from their peers. Such monkeys, even though their fetal life and their first year with their mother was completely normal, fail to show the "double foot-clasp mount" mentioned above, and fail to mount females when they are adults. Thus, although these behaviors are dependent on prenatal exposure to androgens, they also require an environmental factor: contact with playmates. It is as if the sex-specific interactions among juveniles are a necessary intermediary between prenatal organizational effects on the brain and adult sexual behavior. It is interesting that during this long period there is little if any sex difference in the blood levels of testosterone: the hormone is at very low levels throughout childhood in both males and females. Behavior differs between male and female juveniles only because of the greater exposure of the male brain to testosterone before birth and perhaps during the first few months of infancy.

Puberty itself is under direct control of the brain. The key players seem to be the hypothalamic neurons that produce and secrete luteinizing hormone–releasing hormone—the same cells whose role in the luteinizing hormone surge and the menstrual cycle was discussed above. Triggered by some developmental event whose nature is not entirely clear—the attainment of a critical body mass is the most popular candidate—these neurons greatly increase the synthesis and release of LHRH, which in turn induces the increased release of luteinizing hormone and another hormone, follicle-stimulating hormone, from the pituitary gland. These hormones in turn activate the gonads to increase the production of sex steroids, mainly androgens in males, and estrogens and progesterone in females. The raised levels of sex steroids bring about the completion of the sexual differentiation of the body and activate the brain mechanisms of adult sexual behavior.

A rare congenital condition known as Kallmann's syndrome is characterized by two apparently unrelated symptoms: the inability to smell and the delayed onset of puberty. The delayed puberty is caused by the absence or defective function of the LHRH-producing neurons of the hypothalamus, and administration of synthetic LHRH will trigger puberty in the affected individuals. Recent research in animals has shed light on why the two symptoms occur together. It turns out that the LHRH neurons are interlopers in the brain. They do not originate in the lining of the ventricles like other brain neurons. Instead, they originate in the part of the outer surface of the embryonic body that later gives rise to the olfactory mucosa at the back of the nose. They migrate into the brain along the olfactory nerves and take up residence in the hypothalamus as if they were brain natives. This curious and long migration is reminiscent of the lengthy migration of the precursors of the oocytes from the yolk sac to the developing ovary, mentioned in chapter 3. Presumably the defect in Kallmann's syndrome affects all the cells of the primitive olfactory epithelium, both those destined to become olfactory receptors and those destined to migrate into the brain.

In this chapter we have seen that both nature and nurture are at work in the development of sexuality, and that to some extent at least the two factors have to interact during development. The effects of nature are exemplified primarily by the genetically controlled differences in prenatal androgen levels that have such multifarious effects on the sexual development of the body and the brain, including effects on neuron survival, synaptic connections, and neurotransmitter synthesis. The uterine contiguity and maternal stress effects do not exactly come under the category of nurture, but they are certainly environmental effects from the point of view of the developing fetus. Postnatally, we have mentioned the nurture effects of licking behavior in rats and of peer contacts in mon-keys. Still, the emphasis must be on nature. The effects of prenatal hormonal levels are dramatic and long-lasting. While nurture can indeed be shown experimentally to play a significant role, it is much less clear to what extent the range of environments to which individuals are com-monly exposed actually contribute to the diversity of sexual behavior that they exhibit. This theme will be pursued further in chapter 12.

11

In All Suits Like a Man

Sex Differences Beyond Sex

Up to now we have dealt with behavioral traits, and brain systems, that are more or less directly connected with sexual function. Yet there are differences in the mental lives of men and women, and in the brain circuits that underlie them, that extend well beyond the sphere of sex itself. These differences, and their causes, are the subject of this chapter.

It should be stressed at the outset that most of these nonsexual differences between males and females are statistical in nature: there is nearly always a considerable overlap between what is seen in the two sexes, so that it takes measurement of a large number of individuals to be sure that the sex differences are real. This does not take away from the significance of the differences, but it implies that genetic sex is only one of several factors influencing these traits. We shall see in the next chapter that sexual orientation is another such factor. Environmental influences doubtless play a role too: we shall point out some evidence for this.

One sex-differentiated trait is aggressiveness. Among mammals, and certainly among humans, males are generally more aggressive than females. Females are sometimes aggressive too, but their aggressive behavior tends to show itself in particular circumstances such as when their young are threatened. Male aggression can be goal-oriented, as in competition for food, territory, mates, or for position in a hierarchy, but much male aggression seems to be just "for the hell of it."

The greater aggressiveness of males is apparent already in juvenile play behavior—the rough-and-tumble play that, as discussed in the previous chapter, is dependent on prenatal androgen exposure. The increased levels of testosterone from puberty onward are clearly responsible in great part for male-typical aggressiveness in many species. The docility of males castrated before puberty (including human eunuchs) is well known.

One brain region that plays an especially important role in aggressive behavior is the *amygdala*. This structure has been mentioned previously as a source of highly processed sensory information relevant to sexual behavior. The size of a small nut (its name derives from the Greek for almond), the amygdala is located off to the side of the hypothalamus, and a large bundle of axons interconnects the two structures. Like the thalamus and hypothalamus, the amygdala contains several nuclei of distinct though related functions. The common theme that links the nuclei of the amygdala is that they contribute to behaviors that in humans at least have a strong emotional loading: aggression, fear-driven behavior, and sexual behavior. Destruction of the amygdala makes animals unusually docile. In some countries, such as India, bilateral ablation of the amygdala is performed routinely on very aggressive adults and children whose behavior has not responded to other forms of treatment.

The regions of the amygdala that are involved in sexual and aggressive behavior are named the *corticomedial* and *basolateral* nuclei, respectively. The names indicate the positions of the two cell groups within the amygdala. The corticomedial nucleus connects mainly with the medial preoptic area of the hypothalamus. Lesions to this nucleus, in male rats, interfere markedly with the animal's sexual behavior: not only does the rat fail to mount an estrous female, he does not even approach and investigate her. It is as if he is totally deprived of information labeling her as a potential sex partner. The nucleus is larger in male than in female rats and is very rich in androgen receptors.

The basolateral nucleus, on the other hand, is connected primarily with regions further back in the hypothalamus that play a role in aggressive behavior. Lesions of the basolateral nucleus reduce aggressive behavior in both rats and primates. In addition, lesions of this region in juvenile monkeys reduce rough-and-tumble play behavior. It may be that the same neural circuits are involved in rough-and-tumble play and in adult aggression: the change from one form of behavior to the other may be brought about by the increased circulating androgen levels after puberty. The neurons of the basolateral nucleus also possess androgen receptors, although not at the same high levels as are found in the corticomedial nucleus. It is not clear whether the basolateral nucleus is sexually dimorphic.

The aggressiveness shown by females defending their young ("maternal aggression") is brought about by complex interactions of hormonal and sensory events. Increased maternal aggressiveness is one of the signs of the uterine contiguity effect (see chapter 10); thus early androgen exposure can have an organizational influence on this type of aggression just as it does in male aggression. In rodents, the female's aggressiveness increases markedly during the second half of pregnancy under the influence of progesterone, the blood levels of which are high during this time. The mother's aggressiveness decreases when the pups are born, but then increases again to very high levels a day or two later. This postpartum aggression only occurs if the pups are allowed to suckle from the mother, and in fact it is sensory input from the nipples that triggers it. The brain circuits involved are not well understood.

A particularly striking example of the interaction between fetal androgens, aggressiveness and sexual differentiation is the case of the spotted hyena. In this species there is murderous competition between littermates for milk, a competition the mother is helpless to prevent because, except for when they are actually nursing, the pups are housed in narrow tunnels which she cannot enter. To aid them in this fratricidal struggle, the pups are born (like that famous brother-killer, Richard the Third) with fully erupted front teeth. Under the influence of large amounts of androgens secreted by their ovaries and adrenal glands, the female pups are as aggressive as the males, if not more so. As an unwanted by-product of this behavioral masculinization, the external genitalia of the females are also masculinized by the high levels of testosterone: the clitoris is enlarged so much as to resemble the male penis, and it encloses an orifice that has to do the combined duty of urethra, vagina, and birth canal.

Males tend to perform better than females at some tasks that require spatial or visuospatial skills. Male rats, for example, perform better in mazes than do females. Men outscore women (on average) on a variety of spatial tasks. One such task is mental rotation: the subject is shown drawings of a complex object from two different views, and is asked whether or not they are of the same object. To determine the answer the subject must mentally visualize rotating the object from the view seen in one drawing until it matches (or fails to match) the other view. The male superiority at this task is seen already among children. Another commonly used test is the water-level test: the subject is asked to indicate the surface level of some water in a drawing of a tilted flask. Men tend to (correctly) indicate the surface level as horizontal, while women tend to tilt the water level in the same direction as the flask is tilted. Whether this is truly a test of spatial ability or whether it is a test of intuitive-versus-logical thinking, the superior performance by men is dramatic: in one study by Sandra Witelson at McMaster University 92% of the (heterosexual) men but only 28% of the women passed the test.

Conversely, women tend to outperform men on some tests of verbal ability. The differences are less marked than for the spatial tasks, and not all studies have yielded consistent results. The aspect of verbal skill that shows the clearest sex difference is verbal fluency: women are generally better at rapidly producing a set of words that belong to a particular category. The superior verbal abilities shown by women may reflect a difference between the sexes in the degree to which language is a *lateralized* function of the brain. In most individuals of both sexes language is predominantly a function of the left hemisphere. But women tend to have at least *some* representation of language in the right hemisphere also. Perhaps for this reason, women in general recover language better than men do after strokes affecting the left hemisphere.

Are these cognitive differences inborn or learned? It would not be hard to construct an argument for their being learned. One could say that parents encourage their sons to explore their surroundings and play sports, thus training their spatial sense, while girls are encouraged to stay home and read, thus improving their verbal skills. In fact, however, there is some evidence that they are strongly influenced by events prior to birth. Women who were exposed to high levels of androgenizing hormones while they were fetuses, either because they suffered from congenital adrenal hyperplasia or because their mothers were given the synthetic steroid diethylstilbestrol, score better than other women on spatial tests. Similarly, the maze-running performance of female rats that were given androgens around the time of birth is better than that of untreated females. Contrary to expectation, however, androgen-exposed women do not seem to do any worse at verbal tests than control women, and as for rats, their verbal skills are already so poor that no amount of hormone treatment could impair them further.

Another piece of evidence in favor of the idea that sex differences in cognitive skills may be at least partly inborn comes from the study of individuals with the *androgen-insensitivity syndrome*. These are chromosomal males with functioning testes that secrete testosterone. However, they carry a mutation in the gene for the androgen receptor which renders the receptor incapable of recognizing and binding androgens. For this reason it seems to the body as if no androgens are present; the body therefore develops as a female, and the individuals are raised as girls. When Julianne Imperato-McGinley and her colleagues at Cornell University Medical School compared the cognitive skills of these women with those of their normal male and female relatives, they found not only that these women did worse on visuospatial tasks than did their male relatives, they even did worse than their female relatives. The likely explanation for this is that even the low levels of androgens present in normal females during development act to raise spatial abilities above a certain baseline. This baseline performance is seen only in complete absence of androgens or, as with these subjects, a complete insensitivity to any androgens that may be present. By contrast, no differences were noted among between the groups in verbal skills.

There are also structural differences between the brains of males and females outside of the regions directly involved in sexual behavior. First, in species such as humans where males, on average, have bigger bodies, they also have bigger brains. Men's brains are on average 15% bigger than women's. One might expect these sex differences to be most marked for brain regions directly involved in controlling the body (for example, the motor regions of the cerebral cortex) and least marked or absent for regions involved in more abstract tasks where the size of the body is irrelevant. To my knowledge, however, such regional differences have not so far been documented.

Among the individual brain regions showing sexual dimorphism, the most interesting are the *corpus callosum* and the *anterior commissure*. As mentioned in chapter 4, the corpus callosum is the major connection between the left and right hemispheres of the cerebral cortex. Originating as the axons of millions of individual neurons scattered throughout the cerebral cortex, it coalesces as it runs toward the midline within the white matter of the cerebral hemispheres. At the midline it vaults across the fluid-filled gap between the two hemispheres; axons running in the two directions are closely intermingled as they cross this bridge. If one cuts the brain into left and right halves and then looks at the midline structures exposed by the cut, the corpus callosum is especially obvious as a glistening white band that arches over the thalamus and the other deep structures of the brain. The front and back ends of the band (named the *rostrum* and *splenium* of the corpus callosum) are much thicker than the central portion, the *isthmus*. There is an ordering of fibers within the corpus callosum, such that axons originating in the back parts of the cortex (which are mostly visual in function) travel predominantly in the back part of the corpus callosum, the splenium, while axons interconnecting the front regions of the cortex travel in the rostrum. The anterior commissure is, as it were, the corpus callosum's baby sister: it is also an axonal connection between the hemispheres, but it is much smaller. The anterior commissure is the "old" connection between the hemispheres, found in most vertebrates: the corpus callosum was first invented by placental mammals.

Both the corpus callosum and the anterior commissure have been reported to be larger in women than in men. In the case of the corpus callosum, there has been some controversy: some studies report the callosum to be larger in absolute size in women, some report that only certain parts of it, especially the splenium, are larger. In a recent study by Sarah Archibald, William Heindel, and myself, based on brain scans of living men and women, we found the corpus callosum to be about the same size in women and men, but on account of the generally smaller brain size in women the corpus callosum was significantly bigger in women relative to overall brain size. In other words, the corpus callosum occupies a larger fraction of the entire brain volume in women than in men, suggesting that the two cerebral hemispheres are more richly interconnected in women. The anterior commissure has been reported to be larger in absolute size in women than in men, again supporting the idea that women's cerebral hemispheres are more richly interconnected than men's.

It is possible that the stronger interconnection of the two sides of the brain in women has consequences for cognitive processes. It might be related to women's greater verbal fluency and the fact, mentioned above, that language seems to be less completely restricted to the left hemisphere in women. If language, or other functions, have a bilateral representation in the brain, there is that much greater need for connections between the two sides. In fact, Melissa Hines and her colleagues at UCLA have reported that, among normal women, those who score the best on tests of verbal fluency also tend to have the largest splenium of the corpus callosum.

There are also commonly believed to be differences between men and women in traits that are very hard to measure scientifically. It is often said, for instance, and I incline to believe it, that women are generally more "in touch with their feelings" than are men. Since the two hemispheres are thought to differ to some extent in "personality," the left hemisphere being more analytical and verbally expressive, and the right more emotional, artistic, musical, etc., it is not unreasonable to think that a larger corpus callosum and anterior commissure might make an individual better at expressing her or his feelings. Unfortunately, these ideas are too nebulous to test in any rigorous fashion.

12

So Full of Shapes Is Fancy

Sexual Orientation and Its Development

The most remarkable thing about sex is its diversity. Probably no two persons on earth have exactly the same ideas about who or what is sexually attractive or what would be the most appropriate way to consummate this attraction. If we wish to understand sex in biological terms, the basis of this diversity in feelings and behavior must be a central part of our study. Unfortunately, this aspect of sex is so beset by prejudice and ignorance that rational discussion of the topic has, until recently at least, been all but impossible.

One way to categorize people's sexuality is along the dimension of *sexual orientation*. This means the direction of sexual feelings or behavior toward individuals of the opposite sex (heterosexuality), the same sex (homosexuality), or some combination of the two (bisexuality). Much of this chapter will be devoted to this dimension of sexual diversity.

Of course, people's feelings do not always coincide with their behavior. Individuals whose feelings are entirely homosexual may nevertheless, on the basis of religious convictions, a desire to conform, or for other reasons, never put these feelings into practice. Similarly, there are those whose sexual feelings are completely directed to the opposite sex, yet whose sexual activity is largely or entirely homosexual, either because this activity is their livelihood or because, as with prisoners, sexual partners of the opposite sex are not available.

The direction of sexual feelings is undoubtedly more significant, deeper, and less susceptible to change than the direction of sexual behavior. There is good reason, however, to consider both aspects when discussing sexual orientation. Behavior is indisputable and observable; feelings are hidden and only indirectly accessible to study. Behavior is what is studied in animals, therefore animal research bears more directly on human behavior than on human feelings. Lastly, behavior may indicate the existence of feelings that people are unwilling to admit to others or even to themselves.

The terms "heterosexual," "bisexual," and "homosexual" by no means provide a complete description of a person's sexuality. Within all three of these categories, individuals differ greatly in their preferred sexual activities and the roles they prefer to play in them. These differences are particularly evident among gay men and lesbian women. Some of the descriptors that have been used in this context are active/passive, top/bottom, straight-acting/effeminate, butch/femme, and so on. The implication of these labels is that homosexual pairings are generally between two individuals who prefer different gender roles, one preferring the role typical for his or her sex (the "top" gay man and the "femme" lesbian woman) and the other preferring the sex-atypical role (the "bottom" gay man and the "butch" lesbian woman).

There is unquestionably an element of truth in this dichotomy, as anyone who has spent time in the gay and lesbian communities or has read the personal ads in gay or lesbian magazines, is well aware. But it is also an oversimplification. There are certainly some gay men who are markedly effeminate in their general behavior and strongly prefer the receptive role in anal intercourse, and there are some who are very straight-acting, even macho, in their behavior and only take the insertive role in anal intercourse. (Indeed, these latter men sometimes deny that their behavior constitutes homosexuality.) But the preferred sex role is by no means always predictable from the tenor of the individual's general behavior. Even more important, numerous surveys have shown that large numbers of gay men have no strong preference for one or the other genitoerotic role, and freely interchange roles even with the same partner. Furthermore, there are many sexual practices that do not involve distinct "masculine" and "feminine" roles.

What is the distribution of heterosexuality, bisexuality, and homosexuality in the population? The answer to this apparently simple question has foundered on a reef of practical problems: how to obtain a representative sample of the population, how to get them to tell the truth, and how to assess their sexual orientation on the basis of the answers they give.

The most well-known and pioneering efforts in this regard were the studies of Alfred Kinsey and his colleagues in the United States in the 1940s and 1950s. They interviewed many thousands of men and women and asked them about many different aspects of their sexual lives. The major finding, sensational in its time, was the commonness of homosexual behavior: Kinsey calculated that 37% of the male population had at least some overt homosexual experience to the point of orgasm between adolescence and old age, 10% were more or less exclusively homosexual for at least 3 years of their lives, and 4% percent were exclusively homosexual throughout their lives after the onset of adolescence. The figures for women were somewhat lower: 13% of the women interviewed had had some overt homosexual experience to orgasm after adolescence, and 1–3% of unmarried women and less than 0.3% of married women were exclusively homosexual. In Kinsey's data, sexual orientation appeared to be a broad spectrum in which large numbers of individuals fell somewhere between the two extremes.

Kinsey was vehemently attacked, not only by conservatives and religious leaders, but also by other scientists. Margaret Mead, famous for her studies of sexuality in primitive cultures, was an especially persistent critic. She not only attacked the research on technical grounds, she also argued that it should not have been published because it undermined the resolve of young people who were trying to lead "conventional" sex lives. (One hears exactly the same argument used against sex research today, but more frequently from politicians than scientists.) Under these pressures the Rockefeller Foundation discontinued its financial support for Kinsey's research and much of his data was never published. But his two books, *Sexual Behavior in the Human Male* and *Sexual Behavior in the Human Female*, remain among the most-read of any scientific publications: it is hard to find a copy of either book in a library or elsewhere that is not tattered and annotated almost beyond readability. For amidst the cold objectivity and dry statistics lay a message of extraordinary significance: that people's actual sexual behavior does not conform to the norms prescribed by public morality, religion, or the law.

Kinsey's studies were not without their defects. Although he interviewed very large numbers of people, his sampling strategy was quite haphazard by today's standards. For example, he oversampled people who were or had been in prison, and this is believed to have led to a significant exaggeration of the numbers of bisexual individuals in the population. His interviewers relied extensively on leading questions ("When was your first homosexual experience?" rather than "Have you ever had a homosexual experience?"). Also, Kinsey himself was convinced that homosexuality was environmentally determined, and while he apparently did not view it as pathological, he refused to allow lesbians or gay men to work with him. Still, his work did much to open people's eye to the reality of human sexual behavior.

Since Kinsey's time there have been numerous further attempts to assess sexual orientation in both the United States and other countries. Some of these studies have used much more rigorous sampling techniques, akin to those used in political opinion polls. These studies have come up with considerably lower estimates of the prevalence of homosexuality in the population. It is not clear whether the lower numbers are closer to the truth or whether they reflect a failure to elicit honest answers from the interviewees. In any event, the best current "guesstimate" seems to be that about 4–5% of the male population and 2–4% of the female population are predominantly homosexual for a large part of their lives. Further research on this issue is badly needed.

Even less certain is whether there are differences in the incidence of homosexuality in different countries or cultures or in the same culture at different times. Such differences may exist, but what varies most is probably people's attitudes towards homosexuality. These different attitudes can greatly influence the apparent prevalance of homosexuality at different times and places.

I do not know—nor does anyone else—what makes a person gay, bisexual, or straight. I do believe, however, that the answer to this question will eventually be found by doing biological research in laboratories and not by simply talking about the topic, which is the way most people have studied it up to now.

Believing in a biological explanation for sexual orientation is not the same thing as insisting that sexual orientation is inborn or genetically determined. Our entire mental life involves biological processes. We know that our sexual orientation, like our tastes in music and our memory of our last vacation, is engraved in some morphological or chemical substrate in the brain. It is not maintained solely by the brain's actual activity, whether electrical or metabolic. This activity can be brought to a complete stop, for example by cooling the brain to near the freezing point. Yet, once restarted, we regain our original sexual feelings, we still prefer the same composers, and our memories are unimpaired, except for events immediately prior to losing consciousness. So both inborn and environmental factors influence us by influencing the anatomical or chemical structure of the brain.

One of the first people to think about sexual orientation in anything resembling biological terms was the German lawyer Karl Heinrich Ulrichs (1825–1895). Ulrichs, subject of a fine biography by Hubert Kennedy, was the first gay activist. In 1867 he rose before the Congress of German Jurists to demand repeal of the sodomy statutes. Cut off by ridicule and abuse before even reaching the main topic of his speech, Ulrichs' move cost him disgrace and the ruination of his career, and on the face of it achieved nothing for gay rights. Yet his action marked the end of an age in which the legal persecution of homosexual men and women went unchallenged.

In his writings Ulrichs put forward a developmental explanation of homosexuality. He argued that the body and the mind are each programmed to develop along male or female lines, and that a homosexual individual is one in whom bodily development is of one sex, while mental development is of the other. Ulrichs bolstered his theory by the assertion that he, and other gay men, had many feminine traits other than the direction of their sexual drive. Curiously, these traits were not apparent to Ulrichs' friends and acquaintances, who considered him a "regular guy." Yet the existence of these other sex-atypical traits is important to Ulrichs' argument, for otherwise it smacks of tautology: a gay man has a woman's mind simply because being sexually attracted to men is typical of women. Furthermore, Ulrichs' conception, even at a purely descriptive level, would seem to correspond more to what we now call transsexuality than to garden-variety homosexuality, because most gay and lesbian individuals identify strongly with their anatomically defined sex.

In spite of these weaknesses, Ulrichs' ideas have formed the basis for most subsequent thinking and biological research on the topic. I believe that there is an important kernel of truth in his ideas although, a century and more later, this still remains to be proven.

Around the beginning of the twentieth century two major figures, Havelock Ellis and Magnus Hirschfeld, began the objective study of sexual orientation. On the basis of their observations both these men (one straight, one gay) became convinced that homosexuality and heterosexuality were equally normal aspects of human nature that were laid down by some intrinsic mechanisms during early development. Their contributions, however, were overshadowed by the work and writings of Sigmund Freud.

In the earlier part of his career, Freud was quite open to the idea that intrinsic developmental processes might play a significant role in influencing a person's sexual orientation as well as other facets of personality. Later, he came to think of male homosexuality as resulting from a young boy's failure to separate himself from an intense sexual bond with his mother; as a consequence, the boy identifies with her and seeks to reenact (this time playing her role) the relationship that existed between them. As to what might cause this failure of separation, Freud envisaged that it might result from the close-binding nature of the mother, the hostility, weakness, or absence of the father, sibling jealousy, or other factors. Freud saw anal intercourse (a common but by no means universal practice in male homosexuality) as confirming his "failure of development" model of homosexuality, since he believed that all children pass through an "anal phase" before their sexual feelings become focused in their genitals. In regards to homosexuality in women, Freud seems to have envisaged a roughly mirror-image developmental process to the one he postulated for men.

Although he denied this in some of his writings (especially in his well-known letter to an American mother of a gay man), there is no doubt that Freud viewed heterosexuality as the normal adult condition and homosexuality as a pathological state of arrested development caused primarily by defective parenting. This attitude was held even more strongly by his followers, and it invaded the fields of psychiatry and psychology, totally eclipsing the influence of Ellis, Hirschfeld, and others. Of course, thinking of homosexuality as a disease could be considered an advance over thinking of it as a crime or a sin. But in the spirit of medical optimism that has characterized the twentienth century, disease implies curability, and untold thousands of gay men have been subjected to psychoanalysis, castration, testicle grafts, hormone treatments, electric shock therapy, and brain surgery in attempts to "cure" them of their unfortunate condition. As far as I can determine, not one of these treatments ever produced the desired result, but the physical and psychological damage done by them must be counted among the most serious crimes ever committed by the medical profession. Furthermore, the parents of gay men and lesbian women must also be included among the victims of Freudianism: attributing homosexuality to parental behavior, in the context of a generally homophobic society, has been equivalent to burdening them with wholly undeserved blame and guilt.

The observation by Freud and other analysts that gay men tend to recollect their fathers as hostile or distant, and their mothers as unusually close, does seem to have some validity. Surveys of gay men in nonclinical settings support the same conclusion, even though it is far from being a hard-and-fast rule. But, as the psychoanalyst Richard Isay has pointed out, it may well be that Freud confused cause and effect. It is very possible, in other words, that the young pre-homosexual child already exhibits "gay" traits, and that these traits evoke negative reactions from fathers and positive ones from mothers. In support of this interpretation one can cite the cross-cultural studies of the sociologist Frederick Whitam of Arizona State University. Whitam reported that in countries such as Brazil which are relatively tolerant of homosexuality, gay men are less likely to recall their relationships with their fathers as distant or hostile than they are in more homophobic societies such as the United States. It is also possible that these recollections of childhood are not wholly accurate: that they are constructions whose purpose is to screen off unacceptable memories such as a young boy's erotic attachment to his father.

Homosexuality runs in families. Many gay men and lesbian women have at least one brother or sister or other close relative who is also homosexual. From statistical studies (especially one carried out by Richard Pillard and James Weinrich at Boston University) it emerges that having a gay brother increases your own chances of being gay several-fold: about 25% of all the brothers of gay men are themselves gay, whereas in the general male population the incidence of homosexuality is probably under 10%, as mentioned above. The studies on women are less extensive, but it is believed that about 15% of the sisters of lesbian women are themselves lesbian, a figure that is also well above the incidence in the general population. There are conflicting data on whether the grouping of homosexual individuals crosses the sex lines: that is, whether having a gay brother increases a woman's chance of being lesbian, and vice versa. The weight of the evidence is that it does not, or does so only weakly. This suggests that the factors influencing sexual orientation in men may be different from those operating in women. This is reasonable enough, given that "homosexuality" is just a label for two phenomena that are really different things in the two sexes: being attracted to men in one case and being attracted to women in the other.

Such family grouping by itself does not distinguish between the effects of nature and nurture. If parents treated one child in such a way as to make him or her homosexual, they might well treat another child in the same way. More telling evidence for an inborn component comes from the studies of twins, especially from a comparison of monozygotic (identical) twins, who share the same genes, and dizygotic (fraternal) twins, who are no more closely related than non-twin siblings.

Pairs of monozygotic twins, both of whom were homosexual, were described already by Hirschfeld at the turn of the century. Since then there have been a number of studies, some claiming almost total concordance (both twins gay), others noting substantial numbers of discordant pairs (one gay and one straight twin). Two recent studies (one by Michael Bailey of Northwestern University and Richard Pillard; the other by Fred Whitam and colleagues at Arizona State University) have reported that having a gay monozygotic twin makes your own likelihood of being gay about 50–65%, while having a gay dizygotic twin makes your chances of being gay only about 25–30%. In a comparable study of female twins, Bailey, Pillard, and Yvonne Agyei reported that 48% of the monozygotic twin sisters of lesbian women were also lesbian, while only 16% of the dizygotic twin sisters were lesbian, about the same as the rate for non-twin sisters of lesbian women.

These studies are of course beset by problems that might have distorted the estimates of heritability in one direction or another. The subjects who volunteered for the study might not have been representative of the entire population, or the causes of homosexuality among twins might be different from those operating among singletons. Such factors could have inflated the estimates of heritability. Alternatively, the fact that some of the twins studied were quite young might have led to an underestimate of heritability, since some individuals do not acknowledge their own homosexuality till quite late in life.

The best available model for distinguishing inborn from postnatal environmental factors is the case of identical twins separated at birth and raised separately. Unfortunately, such twin pairs are difficult to locate and study, and the additional requirement that at least one of the twins be gay makes the search even harder. Thomas Bouchard and his colleagues at the University of Minnesota have for many years studied twins raised apart. They identified two cases of male identical twins where one of the twins was gay. In one case, the co-twin was also gay. In fact the pair (neither of whom knew he had a twin brother) met after one was mistaken for his twin at a gay bar, and they subsequently became lovers. The other case was more equivocal: one twin considered himself gay, but had had some heterosexual experience, the other considered himself completely heterosexual, but had had a 3-year homosexual relationship as a teenager. The Minnesota group also identified three female pairs where one twin was lesbian. In all three of these cases, the co-twin was entirely heterosexual.

All in all, these twin studies point to a strong but not total genetic influence on sexual orientation in men, and a substantial but perhaps somewhat weaker genetic influence in women. Clearly, some nongenetic factors make a contribution. Ideally, study of the discordant identical twin pairs would allow one to identify these factors, but in practice this has proved very difficult. Identical twins generally are treated very similarly by their parents and siblings, and the life experiences of the two twins do not give obvious clues as to their ultimate sexual orientation. Indeed, sometimes these experiences are the opposite of what one might expect. For example, it has often been claimed that sexual molestation of girls contributes to homosexuality in adulthood. Yet in one discordant female pair in the Minnesota study (one heterosexual, one bisexual) the heterosexual women, and not her co-twin, was sexually molested as a child.

One should bear in mind that nongenetic factors can operate before birth as well as after birth. We have previously discussed examples of such prenatal factors in animals: the effects of maternal stress and uterine contiguity. Even identical twins do not necessarily share an identical prenatal environment: the blood supply of one twin may be better than the other's, for example, and this in turn may lead to a difference in the twins' birth weights.

Also pointing to a genetic factor is a special case, that of men with an extra X chromosome. These XXY individuals are men because, as explained in chapter 3, it is a gene on the Y chromosome that confers maleness; the number of X chromosomes is irrelevant. Nevertheless, the possession of an extra X chromosome does influence development: these individuals tend to be taller and less intelligent than XY men, and their testes fail to produce sperm—the so-called Klinefelter's syndrome. There have been numerous reports over the years of differences in sexual behavior between XXY and XY men, but the interpretation has been problematic because the individuals were often identified through special circumstances such as their being confined to prisons or mental hospitals. A recent U.S.-Danish study solved this problem by "brute force": the researchers simply karyotyped (counted the chromosomes) of every male resident of Copenhagen who filled certain age and height criteria. Out of thousands of men examined, they identified 16 XXY men and compared their sex histories with those of control men matched for height, age, IQ, and socioeconomic status. There was a highly significant excess of homosexuality among the XXY men compared with the control men.

Of course, an extra X chromosome is very uncommon and is certainly not the usual cause of homosexuality. But this study is important in showing unequivocally that genetic factors *can* influence sexual orientation. The exact mechanism by which the extra X chromosome has its effect remains unclear. XXY men have in general slightly lower testosterone levels in their blood than do XY men. It is conceivable that testosterone levels were also lower during a developmental period critical for the determination of sexual orientation. This relates to the "prenatal hormone" theory discussed further below.

Although most individuals do not become conscious of their sexual orientation until puberty or later, there are childhood traits that are to some extent predictive of adult sexual orientation. In general, these could be summarized by saying that children who later become heterosexual tend to have sex-typical childhoods, while children who later become gay or lesbian tend to have sex-atypical childhoods. Boys who are "sissy," dislike rough games or team sports, prefer reading, and so on, have a greater likelihood of becoming gay than other boys. Boys who exhibit strongly sex-atypical traits, such as preferring the company of girls, playing with dolls rather than trucks, and liking to put on girls' or women's clothes, have an even greater likelihood of becoming gay. This is known not just from gay men's recollections of their childhood, but from prospective studies, especially that conducted by Richard Green, a psychiatrist who now works at UCLA Medical School. Green studied markedly "sissy" boys as children and then followed them through to adulthood; the great majority of them eventually became gay or bisexual. It seems that sex-atypical traits are recognizable in some children within the first year or two of life.

From the work of James Weinrich and colleagues at UCSD it appears that gay men who, as adults, have a strong preference for receptive anal intercourse, also have the strongest recollections of sex-atypical childhoods. If this finding is correct, it suggests that these men form a distinct subgroup, for whom their preferred erotic role is in a sense a continuation of a life-long sex-atypical form of self-expression. For gay men who do not have a strong preference for receptive anal sex, the childhood history may be much more conventional. In fact, there is probably substantial overlap in the childhood characteristics of these gay men with those of heterosexual men, some of whom have markedly effeminate traits both in childhood and as adults. Nevertheless, it is well-documented that most gay men, whatever their preferred form of sexual expression, recall *some* sex-atypical feelings or behaviors as children.

For women, the story is similar, though less clear-cut. Lesbian women tend to recollect more unconventional childhoods than heterosexual women, including such traits as being a tomboy, a leader, being unusually active or exploratory, preferring boys' company, boys' clothes, etc. Again, it cannot be automatically assumed that a tomboyish girl will become a lesbian woman—many such girls do not. Nor does every lesbian woman report being tomboyish as a child. But the association between childhood traits and adult sexuality nevertheless exists in a statistical sense. Although it is not well documented in the literature, I would further guess on the basis of my own discussions with lesbian women that those lesbians who are markedly butch (masculine-acting) as adults have the strongest recollections of being tomboyish as children. Unfortunately, no major prospective study of such girls (comparable to Green's study of boys) has been published.

Explicitly sexual feelings or behavior may of course occur during childhood. I am not referring here to activities like thumb-sucking that according to psychoanalysts are at least partially sexual in nature. I mean feelings of being sexually aroused by the sight of others, sexual games, and actual sexual experiences with other children or with adults. People seem to vary a lot in the degree to which they had such feelings or behavior before puberty, or at least in how well they remember them later. But it is striking how closely such childhood sexuality, when it does occur, resembles the person's sexuality as an adult. That is, heterosexual men and women tend to recall childhood sexual feelings directed to the opposite sex, homosexual men and women toward the same sex. Even the details of childhood sexuality often seem uncannily predictive of what follows in adulthood.

A striking example has been described by Fred Whitam. This was a pair of male monozygotic twins, both gay, both fairly effeminate, and both attracted to very masculine "trucker" types of men. As 7-year-old boys, these twins invented a game they named "Chasing Rabbits." They would play naked near the town garbage dump, and, when the garbage trucks came by, they would entice the drivers to chase them into the woods. Some of the drivers did this, and having caught one or both of the children, would bring them back to their cabs and fondle them—the whole point of the game. This story illustrates how sexually active some children can be, and how closely their childhood sexuality can resemble their sexuality as adults.

What is the significance of these childhood traits? First, of course, they mean that even though a person may not become sexually active, or aware of his or her sexual orientation, until puberty or later, nevertheless the factors influencing sexual orientation, or some of these factors, exert their effects well before puberty. To search for the roots of sexual orientation by studying the actual sex experiences of adolescents is, in my view at least, to miss a boat that left port many years earlier.

Beyond that, the existence of childhood gender nonconformity as a predictor of adult homosexuality is very consistent with the idea that adult sexual orientation is influenced by the biological mechanisms of brain development, specifically the sexual differentiation of the brain under the influence of gonadal steroids. In earlier chapters I described some of the evidence that sex-distinct juvenile behavior, both in animals and in humans, is influenced by prenatal interactions between hormones and the brain. The association between childhood behavior and adult sexual orientation suggests that the latter too may be influenced by the same processes. In fact, congenital adrenal hyperplasia not only modifies girls' play and mothering behavior (see chapters 8 and 10), but also increases the likelihood that they will be lesbian or bisexual in adulthood. In addition, men with the XXY chromosome pattern, who as described above are more likely than XY men to have homosexual feelings as adults, also report a significantly greater incidence of sex-atypical traits as children.

Although the connection between childhood behavior and adult sexuality is so striking, both in the general population and in the special cases just described, the exact nature of the connection is unclear. One possibility would be that both traits are independently influenced by the same prenatal developmental events. Another would be that only childhood traits are directly determined during brain differentiation; adult sexuality might, according to this model, result in some way from the childhood behavior. For example, one might imagine that gender-nonconformist behavior as a child leads to parental reactions (e.g., rejection of a boy by his father) that are necessary for the subsequent development of homosexuality. This would be a loop through the environment analogous to the parental licking behavior in rats, described in chapter 10. This issue is of some relevance because, if this second model is correct, it would imply that in spite of the inborn influences on sexual orientation, the effect of these forces could be modified by modifying the environmental loop (in the example cited, by persuading the father to accept his son's femininity instead of rejecting it). The jury is still out on this issue, although the limited evidence available suggests that in fact the two phenomena, childhood behavior and adult sexuality, may be separately induced by prenatal events rather than being two links in a single causal chain.

As adults, homosexual and heterosexual individuals differ in more than simply who they like to have sex with. Some of these differences support the idea that the brains of homosexual individuals develop in a sex-atypical fashion, as originally suggested by Ulrichs. Other differences may simply reflect the very different life circumstances that straight and gay people face.

In the previous chapter I mentioned that men, on average, tend to score higher than women on certain tests of spatial ability and lower on some tests of verbal ability. Several studies have compared the performance of gay and straight men on such tasks. The findings generally are that gay men tend to score like heterosexual women, or somewhere between the typical scores of heterosexual women and heterosexual men. Most strikingly, gay men's performance at the mental rotation and water-level tasks (see chapter 11) is on average closer to that of women than that of heterosexual men. It is less clear whether gay men have an equivalent superiority in tests of verbal skills: even the differences between the sexes in these tasks are rather small, and the studies that have looked for differences with sexual orientation have yielded inconsistent results.

Another relevant trait is handedness, a complex trait associated with lateralization of cerebral function. The general tendency among both men and women is of course to use the right hand preferentially for a wide variety of tasks. For tasks requiring both hands, the left hand is generally assigned the simpler, stabilizing role (for example, holding a jam-jar while the right hand unscrews the lid). Cheryl McCormick and her colleagues have reported that both gay men and lesbian women are less consistently right-handed, tending to either use their left hands preferentially or, more commonly, to do some tasks with the right hand, some with the left. This difference probably does not result from any parental or educational influence, because the task which is most culturally influenced—writing—shows the least difference in handedness between homosexual and heterosexual people.

The apparent tendency of lesbians and gay men to be less consistently right-handed than heterosexual people suggests that their cerebral functions may less strongly lateralized. There is in fact some direct evidence to support the idea that the cerebral functions of gay men are more symmetrically distributed to the left and right hemispheres than they are in straight men. In terms of causation, though, these observations are puzzling, because, if prenatal hormones are at work here, one would expect opposite effects in gay men and lesbian women. McCormick and her colleagues have suggested that left-handedness is caused by unusually *high* levels of androgens in female fetuses, but by unusually *low* levels of androgens in male fetuses. Although this would explain the results, it is an unsatisfying theory because it demands further explanations of how these opposite effects occur in the two sexes.

Of course, the traits that really interest people are those that color their social interactions, affect their choice of occupation, and so on. These traits have not really been subject to scientific study. Even the question of whether certain occupational fields attract higher- or lower-than-average numbers of gays or lesbians is very difficult to answer, because homosexual individuals are much more accepted, and hence are more open about their sexuality, in some fields than in others. Still, I think that most people would agree that there are subsets of gays and lesbians who are markedly sex-atypical in behavior, skills and interests and who gravitate to occupations where these traits are of value. Jobs requiring leadership and organizational skills; mechanical, electrical, and transportation jobs; athletic and strongly physical occupations; all seem to be especially attractive to a subset of lesbian women. Jobs requiring creative or caring traits—design, writing, dance, theater, nursing, and so on—seem especially attractive to some gay men. But beyond these subsets there are large numbers of gays and lesbians who occupy, often fairly invisibly, the same niches in society that are filled by straight men and women.

On the whole it appears that sex-atypical traits are more uniformly seen in children destined to become gay or lesbian than in adults who *are* gay or lesbian. It is striking that even very "straight-acting" gay men, for example, tend to recall at least some sissiness or other sex-atypical traits from their childhood. One possible explanation for this would be that the increases in levels of androgens and estrogens at puberty stimulate the development of sex-typical traits that had been dormant in these individuals as children. Alternatively, the relentless pressures exerted by society on adolescents may force them to conform more closely to what is expected of their sex.

One life experience that gays and lesbians share is the experience of becoming aware of their own sexuality, accepting it in spite of so much contrary pressure from parents, schools, and society in general, and becoming open about it to others. This total experience—"coming out"—must profoundly influence the mind of every homosexual individual. It seems likely that some traits that characterize many gays and lesbians, especially a distrust of authority and an unusual ability to empathize with others, result at least in part from this experience. If, in some utopian society of the future, the negative pressures on gays and lesbians disappear, it will be interesting to see whether or not these traits disappear with them.

Are there differences in the anatomical or chemical structure of the brain between homosexual and heterosexual individuals? As I stated at the beginning of the chapter, the answer to this question must in principle be yes, because a person's sexual orientation remains unaltered after all brain activity and metabolism have been temporarily halted. So the practical question is: Are the structural differences scattered through a million widely dispersed, anonymous synapses in the cerebral cortex (as the structural differences representing preference for different musical composers presumably are) or are they concentrated at a key location, where they so dominate the cellular landscape as to make themselves evident to an anatomist's inspection?

My own research suggests that there is at least one such key location, the medial preoptic region of the hypothalamus. As you will recall from chapter 9, this region of the brain is believed to be involved in the regulation of male-typical sexual behavior, and it contains at least four small groups of neurons termed the interstitial nuclei of the anterior hypothalamus (INAH). One of these, named INAH 3, is bigger on average in men than women. The others either show no sex differences (INAH 1 and 4) or show equivocal differences that may be limited to certain age ranges (INAH 2). I obtained the brains of gay men (all of whom had died of AIDS) as well as the brains of heterosexual men who had also died of AIDS (these were intravenous drug abusers) and of presumably heterosexual men who had died of a variety of other causes. In addition, I obtained the brains of several women, presumably heterosexual ("presumably" means simply on the basis of the preponderance of heterosexual women in the population: a woman's sexual orientation is rarely if ever noted in her medical records). I was not able to obtain the brains of any women known to have been lesbian.

I processed and analyzed the hypothalamic tissue from these brains "blind," that is, not knowing which specimen came from which group of subjects. After decoding the results, I obtained two significant results. First, INAH 3 was on average two- to threefold bigger in the presumed heterosexual men (whether or not they died of AIDS) than in the women. This result confirmed that of Laura Allen and colleagues at UCLA. Second, in the gay men INAH 3 was on average the same size as in the women, and two to three times smaller than in the straight men. It should be emphasized that these differences were in the *averages:* some of the women and gay men had a large INAH 3, and some of the presumed heterosexual men had a small one. None of the other three nuclei showed any differences between groups.

This finding suggests that gay and straight men may differ in the central neuronal mechanisms that regulate sexual behavior. Although the data described only the size of the nuclei, not the numbers of neurons within each nucleus, it is very likely that there are fewer neurons in INAH 3 of gay men (and women) than in straight men. To put an absurdly facile spin on it, gay men simply don't have the brain cells to be attracted to women.

Several important qualifications have to be made. All the gay men in my sample died of AIDS. Was the disease rather than their sexual orientation responsible for the small size of INAH 3? After all, we know that AIDS and its complications can devastate the brain. My reasons for thinking that the disease was not responsible were fivefold. First, the control group of AIDS patients who were heterosexual had a large INAH 3. Second, none of the other three nuclei showed differences between groups, as they might well have done if the disease was destroying neurons nonselectively in this region of the brain. Third, there was no correlation between the length of the patients' illness, or the complications that occurred, and the size of INAH 3. Fourth, there were no dying cells, inflammatory reactions, or other signs of a pathological process at work. Lastly, after publication of my study I obtained the brain of one gay man who died of a disease other than AIDS (he died of lung cancer). I examined this brain "blind" along with three other brains from presumably heterosexual men of similar ages. Already during the analysis I correctly guessed which was the hypothalamus of the gay man; INAH 3 was less than half the size of the nucleus in the other three men.

Even if, as I believe, AIDS was not the reason for the difference in the size of INAH 3, the use of brains from AIDS patients does raise other problems. Are gay men who die of AIDS representative of gay men as a whole, or are they atypical, for example in preferring receptive anal intercourse (the major risk factor in homosexual sex) or in having unusually large numbers of sexual partners (another risk factor)? It is difficult to answer these questions decisively. However, HIV infection is now so widespread in the gay community that it is unrealistic to imagine a group to be highly atypical simply because they died of AIDS.

To many people, finding a difference in brain structure between gay and straight men is equivalent to proving that gay men are "born that way." Time and again I have been described as someone who "proved that homosexuality is genetic" or some such thing. I did not. My observations were made only on adults who had been sexually active for a considerable period of time. It is not possible, purely on the basis of my observations, to say whether the structural differences were present at birth, and later influenced the men to become gay or straight, or whether they arose in adult life, perhaps as a result of the men's sexual behavior.

In considering which of these interpretations is more likely, one is thrown back on the animal research discussed in earlier chapters. As described in chapter 10, the sexually dimorphic nucleus of the medial preoptic area in rats (which may or may not correspond to INAH 3 in humans) is highly susceptible to modification during a critical period that lasts for a few days before and after the rat's birth. After this time, it is difficult to change the size of the nucleus by any means. Even castrating adult rats (which removes the rat's source of androgens and greatly impairs the rat's sexual behavior) has at most a very slight effect on the size of the nucleus. If the same is true for INAH 3 in humans, it would seem likely that the structural differences between gay and straight men come about during the initial period of sexual differentiation of the hypothalamus. If this is the case, it is possible that these differences play some role in determining a person's sexual orientation. However, we cannot exclude the possibility that in humans, with their longer lifespan and better developed cerebral cortex, gross changes in the size of INAH 3 might come about as a result of adult behavior.

The ideal experiment would of course be to measure the size of INAH 3 in newborn infants by some scanning technique, to wait twenty years, and then to inquire about their sexual orientation. If the size of the nucleus at birth were to any extent predictive of the person's ultimate sexual orientation, one could argue more strongly that the size of the nucleus might play some kind of causative role. This experiment is not possible, at the moment at least, as scanning techniques capable of imaging INAH 3 in living people do not yet exist.

In the rat research, the major factor influencing the size of the sexually dimorphic nucleus has been shown to be the levels of circulating androgens, which act on the neurons of the nucleus during the critical period to promote their survival. This suggests two possible developmental mechanisms by which the different size of INAH 3 in gay and straight men might come about. One would be that there are differences between "gay" and "straight" fetuses in the levels of circulating androgens during the critical period for the development of INAH 3. The other would be that the levels of androgens are the same, but that the cellular mechanisms by which the neurons of INAH 3 respond to the hormones are different. These possibilities will be discussed further below.

More recently, another difference in brain structure between gay and straight men has been described, this time by Allen and Gorski at UCLA. They found differences in the anterior commissure, which, as described in chapter 11, is an axonal connection between the left and right sides of the cerebral cortex and is generally larger in women than men. Allen and Gorski's finding (which like my work was made on autopsied brains, many from AIDS patients) was that the anterior commissure is on average larger in gay men than in straight men. In fact they found it to be larger in gay men even than in women, but after correction for overall brain size the size of the structure was about the same in gay men and in women. (As in my study, Allen and Gorski were unable to determine the sexual orientation of the women from their medical records; presumably the majority of them were heterosexual.)

This finding is interesting for several reasons. First, it strengthens the notion that the brains of gay and straight men are indeed different. Second, it may relate to some of the cognitive differences mentioned above: if cerebral functions are less strongly lateralized in gay men than in straight men, there may be greater need to interconnect the two hemispheres. Finally, the very fact that the anterior commissure is *not* involved in the regulation of sexual behavior makes it highly unlikely that the size differences *result* from differences in sexual behavior. Much more probably, the size differences came about during the original sexual differentiation of the anterior commissure, either under the direct influence of gonadal steroids or as a consequence of developmental events in the cortical regions that it interconnects. Thus, whatever the functional significance of the size of the commissure may be, it may serve as an independent label for processes that went forward differently in "gay" and "straight" fetuses or young children.

Unlike INAH 3, which is far too small to be imaged in a living person's brain by any available scanning technique, the anterior commissure can be seen, although not terribly clearly, in magnetic resonance images (MRI scans). Modest improvements in technique might allow the commissure to be measured accurately in living persons. This would allow the issue of brain structure and sexual orientation to be extended to women, and it would also allow one to obtain a detailed sex history, including details of preferred erotic roles, childhood characteristics, and so on, from the same individuals whose brain structures were measured.

The other major connection between the two cerebral hemispheres, the corpus callosum, is also sexually dimorphic, being relatively larger in women than in men (see chapter 11). In a preliminary study in which I and my colleagues at UCSD have been involved, we failed to find significant differences in the size or shape of the corpus callosum between gay and straight men. This issue needs to be investigated further, but it may well be that the corpus callosum mediates sex-differentiated functions that are not atypical, or not markedly so, in gay men.

One scientist who has been particularly wedded to the notion that sexual orientation depends on a prenatal interaction between sex hormones and the brain is the German endocrinologist Gunther Dörner. Dörner claimed to find evidence for this idea in the hormonal responses of gay and straight men to injections of estrogens. As mentioned in chapter 10, female rats respond to such injections with a surge in the secretion of luteinizing hormone from the pituitary gland, while male rats do not. This difference is caused by functional differences in the part of the hypothalamus that regulates pituitary function, and these in turn are brought about by differences in levels of androgens during a critical developmental period. According to Dörner, gay men respond to estrogen injections with a female-like surge in luteinizing hormone secretion, while straight men do not. He has argued that gay men, during some point in fetal life, were exposed to unusually low levels of androgens, which allowed these hypothalamic circuits to develop in a female-typical direction.

Dörner's claim has not held up well. Of three attempts to replicate the finding, one provided partial replication and two failed to confirm it at all. Furthermore, it now seems that the sex difference in the luteinizing hormone response, which is so characteristic of rats, may not exist in humans or other primates at all. Another blow to his theory comes from the women with congenital adrenal hyperplasia, who as described earlier are exposed to high levels of androgens during fetal life and show evidence of partial brain masculinization in terms of childhood behavior and sexual orientation in adulthood. These women have no disturbance of reproductive function, even though such disturbance would have been expected if a key element in the endocrine control of their menstrual cycle were masculinized.

Nothing daunted, Dörner has gone on to offer an explanation for the proposed differences in prenatal hormone levels of gay and straight men, an explanation that also derives from research on rats. Dörner has proposed that maternal stress is a key factor in the etiology of male homosexuality. As described in chapter 10, stress to pregnant rats toward the end of their pregnancy produces male offspring who show unusually low levels of male-typical sexual behavior and (more equivocally) in-creased levels of female-typical behavior, especially in the frequency of lordosis when paired with a stud male. Dörner claimed to find two pieces of evidence that this is relevant to human sexual orientation. First, he cites reports that the frequency of homosexuality is higher among men born during the stressful period during and just after the Second World War than among men born during peacetime. Secondly, he claims to find a greater incidence of stressful events during the pregnancies of women whose sons eventually became gay than in those of women whose sons became straight.

Both these pieces of evidence are fairly weak. First, it is very difficult to obtain reliable data about the relative frequency of homosexuality in different populations (different age groups in this case). Second, there are many other differences between war and peace years besides the level of stress. If one is thinking in Freudian terms, for example, one can appeal to the greater likelihood of fathers' being absent during wartime. Finally, gay and straight men may differ in what they were told by their mothers about their pregnancies or how they remember or interpret what they were told. In an attempt to get around this problem, Michael Bailey and his colleagues at Northwestern University interviewed women who had had at least one gay and one straight son. The women did not report any excess of stressful events during the pregnancies that gave rise to gay sons.

All in all, the evidence for the idea that prenatal stress is a major cause of homosexuality in men seems very weak. Of course, I may be biased away from believing that something as cool as homosexuality could be caused by something as uncool as stress. Dörner's hypothesis does at least deserve further study.

Although Dörner's specific theories have not held up well, his basic idea—that homosexuality, like heterosexuality, results at least in part from specific interactions between androgenic sex hormones and the brain during development—is one that I share. As mentioned above, there are basically two ways in which these interactions could differ between gay and straight individuals: either the hormones themselves are present at different levels, being unusually low in fetuses destined to become gay men and unusually high in fetuses destined to become lesbian women, or else the receptors and other cellular mechanisms that respond to the hormones are different.

In favor of the notion that different hormone levels can play a role are several points. First, this is the presumed mechanism for the increased incidence of homosexuality in women with congenital adrenal hyperplasia, since this condition definitely does cause increased androgen levels during fetal life and does not, as far as we know, cause any intrinsic differences in the brain that could otherwise explain the effect. (One cannot rule out the possibility, however, that the greater likelihood of homosexual feelings in these women is an indirect effect, such as a psychological reaction to the possession of partially androgenized genitalia.) Second, there have been reports, although the data are not overwhelmingly persuasive, that some lesbian women show signs of masculinization of the body, for example in skeletal anatomy. If so, this might be interpreted as further evidence for the presence of high androgen levels at some time during development.

Against this notion is the relative specificity of the effect. By and large, the bodies of heterosexual and homosexual individuals are remarkably similar. Even the brains of homosexual individuals are by no stretch of the imagination fully sex-reversed. We see evidence for that in the preservation of sex-typical gender identity in lesbians and gay men. Another trait that is not generally sex-reversed is the tendency of men to seek more different sex partners than do women. This tendency has its origin in the fact that males are biologically capable of having more offspring than are females (see chapter 2), and it is seen in many species besides our own. According to several surveys, gay men have, on average, many times the number of different partners that lesbian women do. If anything, in fact, this sex difference is exaggerated among homosexual men and women, because gay men, unlike heterosexual men, are not constrained by women's reluctance to have sex with them. Given the existence of these (and probably many other) traits that are not sex-atypical in homosexual individuals, the attempt to explain differences in sexual orientation solely in terms of differences in prenatal hormone levels, as Dörner has attempted to do, requires that there be some very precise window of time in which sexual orientation, but not other aspects of sexual differentiation, is determined.

There is much to recommend the other alternative, namely that there are intrinsic, genetically determined differences in the brain's hormone receptors or in the other molecular machinery that is interposed between circulating hormones and their actions on brain development. First, this would provide a mechanism that involves hormone-induced brain differentiation but which does not require there to be differences in the actual levels of hormones. Second, since there are several different receptors involved (including the androgen receptor, the estrogen receptor, and at least two "estrogen-related" receptors), there is opportunity for selective effects on different brain systems.

This is of course mere speculation at present. But it is not unrealistic to expect a gene or genes influencing sexual orientation to be identified within the next few years, since there are at least three laboratories in the United States alone that are working on the topic. If such genes are found, it will be possible to ask where, when, and how these genes exert their effects, and hence to gain a much more basic understanding of the biological mechanisms that make us straight or gay. Of course such work, like all the research currently devoted to the human genome, carries with it the likelihood of major social consequences: the revision of the public's views about the nature of homosexuality, and the development of screening tests that might give an indication of whether a person (or fetus) is more or less likely to be (or become) gay. All science fiction at present, but perhaps not so far off from becoming scientific reality. Certainly it is not too early to begin thinking about what should or should not be done with this kind of information.

If there are genes that influence people to become homosexual, why do such genes exist and why have they been perpetuated? A number of sociobiologists, including G. E. Hutchinson, E. O. Wilson, J. D. Weinrich, and Michael Ruse, have speculated on this issue, and the following discussion is based on their writings.

On the face of it, evolutionary processes would strongly select against a gene that induced nonprocreative sexual behavior. One possibility is that, during much of human evolution, societal pressures forced men and women to procreate regardless of their sexual orientation. If this was the case, "gay genes" might be maintained because of some other, beneficial traits associated with homosexuality (say increased verbal ability), or because homosexual behavior itself confers some benefit, for example by promoting mutually beneficial cooperation between persons of the same sex.

On the whole, this explanation seems to me unlikely. There is evidence even from preliterate societies that homosexuality is associated with decreased reproduction. Given the intense selection pressures that act on sexual behavior, it is improbable that a lack of sexual attraction to the opposite sex could be sufficiently compensated by purely social forces.

In chapter 2 I alluded to the sociobiological theory of kin selection as a potential explanation for much counterintuitive behavior among animals. It is possible that homosexuality should be viewed in this light. According to this notion, gay genes reduce the direct reproductive success of the individual possessing them, but cause that individual to promote the reproductive success of his or her close relatives. As a specific example, let us think of a man who would otherwise have fathered two children, but on account of his gay genes fathered none. If this man promoted the reproductive interests of his siblings to the extent that they successfully reared four more children than they otherwise would have done, his genes have had the same reproductive success as if he had had two children of his own, because his siblings' children are half as closely related to himself as his own children are. If the gay man does have some direct reproductive success (fathering one child, for example) then of course he only has to help his siblings produce two extra children for his gayness to be "worthwhile."

It is not hard to think of ways in which a gay man might help his siblings produce and successfully rear extra children. The main problem is that this theory does not account for homosexuality, it only accounts for the lack of heterosexuality. To put it crudely, why do gay men waste so much time cruising each other, time that according to this theory would be better spent baby-sitting their nephews and nieces?

Another theory is the so-called "sickle-cell" model for homosexuality. Sickle-cell anemia is a recessive trait: the disease occurs in individuals that are homozygous for the sickle-cell gene, that is, carry copies of it on both homologous chromosomes. Individuals who are heterozygous (i.e., carry just one copy of the gene) do not suffer from the disease, but have slight differences in their red blood cells that confer a resistance to malaria. In areas where malaria is endemic, this advantage to the heterozygous individuals is sufficient to keep the gene in the population. The homozygous condition is just an unwanted by-product, occurring in some of the offspring of matings between heterozygous individuals. The same could be true of a gay gene: it might be preserved in the population because individuals who are heterozygous for the gene, besides not being gay, have some other advantage that improves their reproductive success. This theory, which brands gay men and lesbian women as the losers in a genetic roulette game, may not appeal to many gay men or lesbian women—it certainly doesn't appeal to me—but it nevertheless has some plausibility.

A final possibility is that gay genes *are* in fact deleterious from the point of view of reproductive success, and do tend to get eliminated from the population, but that for some reason the variant genes are re-created at a high rate, so that the genes that are eliminated are replaced by new ones. To evaluate this possibility would require identifying the genes that are involved.

To sum up this chapter, I should emphasize first that the factors that determine whether a person becomes heterosexual, bisexual, or homosexual are still largely unknown. Yet there are indications that sexual orientation is strongly influenced by events occuring during the early developmental period when the brain is differentiating sexually under the influence of gonadal steroids. From family and twin studies, it is clear that genes play a major role, but it remains to be seen whether these genes operate by influencing the level of sex steroids before birth, by influencing the way in which the brain responds to these steroids, or by other means. Environmental factors must also play a role: these could include maternal stress or other environmental influences occurring prenatally, parental and sibling interactions during childhood, or social and sexual interactions at adolescence or in adulthood. None of the proposed nongenetic factors are as yet well supported by scientific evidence. Given the evidence that some brain structures differ between gay and straight individuals and that childhood traits are to some extent predictive of a person's sexual orientation in adulthood, it would seem that environmental factors operating very early in life are better candidates than those operating later. Further progress in this field will most likely come from the identification of the genes that influence sexual orientation, and the mechanisms by which these genes exert their effects. Once these mechanisms have been clarified, it will be much easier to study how environmental processes can interact with them to modify the final outcome.

13

Wrapped in a Woman's Hide

Gender Identity and Transsexuality

Gender identity is the subjective sense of one's own sex. Most individuals, whether heterosexual or homosexual, identify as male or female in concordance with their anatomical sex. Thus one might be tempted to think that one's gender identity results from a lifetime's experience of having male or female genitalia, reinforced by the teachings and social pressure of parents, siblings, and society at large. This seems not to be the whole story, however. Rather, there appears to be a representation of one's sex in the brain whose development is at least partially independent of life experiences. The evidence for this—quite tentative at this point, to be sure—comes from the study of two types of individuals: transsexuals and individuals with genetic errors of metabolism.

Transsexuals are individuals who believe that they really belong to the sex opposite to that indicated by their genitalia. Although there is considerable diversity among transsexuals, there is a core group who are characterized by a coherent set of features. In childhood they are strongly gender-nonconformist. In adulthood, their personalities are highly sex-atypical as measured by a variety of psychological tests. A transsexual man who belongs to this core group has an aversion to his own penis, especially to the use of the penis in sexual activity. He wishes to live and be treated as a woman. He is sexually attracted to heterosexual men. He seeks and often undergoes hormone treatment and reconstructive surgery to change his body as far as possible into that of a woman. He does not show evidence of generalized psychological disturbance. A transsexual woman belonging to this core group exhibits the mirror-image traits.

Beyond this core group, which forms a substantial fraction of those people who request sex-reassignment surgery, there are other transsexual men and women who do not exhibit all these features. Some do derive sexual pleasure from the use of their genitalia. Some are sexually attracted to individuals of the opposite sex. Some do have evidence of psychological disturbance. And some seem intermediate between transsexual and homosexual or transvestite.

So far, the search for biological markers in transsexual men and women has been inconclusive. There have been no reports of sex-atypical brain structures in transsexuals, and while there have been reports of a number of sex-atypical endocrinological markers (such as raised testosterone levels in transsexual women, and an atypical luteinizing hormone response to estrogen in transsexual men), most of these findings have been contradicted by other studies. Nor is there as yet any substantial evidence for a genetic component to transsexuality.

In spite of the lack of such markers, the very existence of transsexuality speaks strongly, in my view, for the notion that gender identity is not necessarily determined by life experiences. For most "core" transsexuals there simply is no history of traumatizing experiences, relationships, or illnesses that could possibly explain such a radical departure from conventionality. And transsexuals do not appear to be mentally ill. There is the world of difference between a man who insists he is a woman and one who insists he is Jesus Christ reincarnated: the latter betrays his insanity with every sentence he utters, while the former is so obviously sane that he can often persuade a surgeon to cut off his penis. I feel confident that biological markers for transsexuality will eventually be identified. When these are found, they may well help us understand the developmental mechanisms that underlie gender identity.

In the 1960s John Money (later joined by Anke Ehrhardt) studied the development of gender identity in individuals who, on account of congenital adrenal hyperplasia, were born with ambiguous genitalia. They reported that gender identity depended on the sex of rearing: bringing up such a child as a girl would produce an adult with female gender identity, and vice versa. The force of their conclusion was weakened, however, by the fact that the actual hormonal status of the individuals, either pre- or postnatally, was not examined; it is therefore not at all clear that the individuals raised as boys and those raised as girls really had comparable hormonal exposure. Furthermore, the sex of rearing was often reinforced by appropriate hormonal treatment, especially at puberty.

As a further bolster to the notion of the predominant role of nurture in the development of gender identity, Money and Ehrhardt described the remarkable case of a pair of identical male twins, one of whom suffered an accidental destruction of the penis during circumcision. This child was subsequently castrated, surgically reconstructed as a girl, and raised as a girl by her parents. Money and Ehrhardt reported that the mother described this child as being much more feminine in many ways than her genetically identical brother. This case is still cited in textbooks as evidence for the influence of environmental factors on gender identity. The fact of the matter, however, is that the girl was always tomboyish and difficult to control, even by her mother's admission. Furthermore, the objectivity of the mother's account has to be seriously questioned, given her natural desire to believe that the sex-reassignment was a wise decision. In any case, the child was apparently lost to follow-up long before puberty, and what has been heard of her since suggests that she has not successfully adopted to a female gender identity. It should be said, by the way, that Money and Ehrhardt later came to place less emphasis on rearing conditions in the development of gender identity and sex-related traits than they did at the time of the studies just mentioned.

Evidence pointing in quite a different direction comes from studies of the individuals suffering from the very rare congenital condition, briefly mentioned in chapter 3, known as *5-alpha-reductase deficiency*. This story began with the discovery, in three remote villages in the Dominican Republic, of a number of individuals who apparently changed sex, from female to male, at puberty. Born with female-like external genitalia, they were raised as girls. At puberty, however, breasts failed to develop. Instead, the clitoris enlarged greatly to resemble a small penis, the voice deepened, facial hair appeared, and the body became muscular like a man's.

These individuals, who were all interrelated, were studied by Julianne Imperato-McGinley of Cornell University Medical School, and a number of colleagues. They found that skin cells from the affected individuals had a greatly reduced ability to convert testosterone into the much more potent androgen dihydrotestosterone. The enzyme responsible for the conversion, known as 5-alpha-reductase, was defective. More recently the gene coding for the enzyme has been located and sequenced by the same group, and they have identified the coding errors that are responsible for the defect in the enzyme. The syndrome is recessive: a person must have defective genes on both homologous chromosomes to show the syndrome, since even a single normal gene produces enough functional enzyme to get the job done.

As you will recall from chapter 3, it is the conversion of testosterone to dihydrotestosterone that permits the external genitalia to differentiate in the male direction during a developmental period when testosterone levels are fairly low. The internal genitalia and the brain, however, do not depend on this conversion: they are responsive to testosterone itself. Thus in 5-alpha-reductase–deficient individuals who are genetic males the internal genitalia and the brain develop in a normal male-typical direction.

In spite of being brought up as girls, nearly all of the affected individuals readily assumed male gender identity when their bodies masculinized. They put on men's clothes, adopted men's activities, developed sexual relationships with women, and in every way considered themselves male.

Another kinship with the same disorder was discovered by D. C. Gajdusek among the Simbari Anga people in the Eastern Highlands of Papua New Guinea. These people have a radically different culture from that of the Dominican Republic kinship: after male initiation rites (prior to puberty) the two sexes are kept rigorously separate, and ritualized oral sex occurs between men from puberty until premarital age. In spite of this barrier between the sexes, most of the affected individuals changed their gender identities from female to male at puberty, albeit with much turmoil.

In both communities, the syndrome eventually became well known, and as a result many of the affected individuals were recognized by careful inspection of the genitalia at birth or soon thereafter, and were raised as boys or as girls who were expected to change sex. From our point of view, however, the significant individuals are those who were raised unambiguously as girls, before the syndrome became apparent. The fact that these individuals adopted male gender identity at puberty suggests that prenatal exposure of the brain to testosterone, combined with the normal activational events of male puberty, overrides any effect of rearing in the determination of adult gender identity.

Because of its subjective nature, gender identity and its development cannot readily be studied in animals. It will therefore be very difficult to pin down the brain circuits and biological mechanisms that are involved. The continued study of transsexuals offers the best hope of progress in this field.

Epilogue
Two Artificial Gods

Sexual orientation and gender identity are just two aspects of human sexuality. Beyond these is a whole realm of diversity. In terms of sexual desires, for example, some people are attracted to mature or older partners, some to young adults, some to children. Some go for skinny, some for fat. Some are turned on by candlelight and soft music, others by whips and abuse. Some are aroused by animals, some by motorbikes, some by corpses. Some like sex in groups, for others the ultimate sex object is their own body. There are even people who never experience sexual feelings of any kind.

One can argue endlessly about what constitutes "normal" sexuality and what should be defined as aberrant or even criminal. But science can only describe what is out there and attempt to discover how it got that way. For the attributes of sexual life just mentioned, little or nothing is known about what generates them, so there is little point in discussing them in detail in a book of this kind. It is likely that life experiences play a significant role in molding the intimate details of a person's sexual drive. Yet even here the potential for inborn differences should not be ignored. We know, for example, that food preferences are influenced by genetic factors; there is no reason why the same should not be true for preferences in sexual life.

Undoubtedly, the future will bring major progress in our understanding of the mechanisms and development of sexuality. The most promising area for exploration is the identification of genes that influence sexual behavior and the study of when, where, and how these genes exert their effects. Given the explosive rate at which the fields of molecular genetics and neurobiology are expanding, it is inevitable that the perception of our own nature, in the field of sex as in all attributes of our physical and mental lives, will be increasingly dominated by concepts derived from the biological sciences.

As emphasized earlier, thinking about the mind in biological terms is not the same thing as believing that all mental traits are genetically determined, since even environmental and cultural influences on the mind operate through biological mechanisms. Furthermore, we have reviewed plenty of evidence in this book that, strong as the influence of genes may be, they do not fully account for the diversity that we see around us. In rats, position in the uterus and maternal stress can influence, through hormonal channels, the animals' sexual behavior in adulthood. Mother-offspring interactions, typified by the anogenital licking behavior in rats, contribute to the development of sex-typical behavior patterns. In monkeys, the infant's interaction with siblings and playmates plays a vital role in the development of its later sexual behavior. In humans, we are not sure what the relative importance of these various nongenetic factors may be, but in sum they must play an important role. The clearest evidence for this comes from the study of monozygotic twins. Though they resemble each other in so many ways, they are not identical: they can differ in something as basic as their sexual orientation, for example. So nature alone, or nurture alone, cannot provide an adequate explanation for our sexual individuality.

The ultimate challenge will be to establish how the genetic differences among individuals interact with environmental factors to produce the diversity that exists among us. But to approach this goal, it will be necessary first to reject the notion of the tabula rasa—the idea, propounded by Locke, that the mind of the newborn child is a blank slate on which experience is free to write whatever it will. In reality, our range of individual development is defined and limited by what we are born with. Like waterlilies, we swing to and fro with the currents of life, yet our roots moor us each to our own spot on the river's floor.

Afterword

Shortly after the publication of this book in 1993, a major advance in the study of sexual orientation was reported by researchers at the National Institutes of Health in Washington, D.C. This group, led by molecular biologist Dean Hamer, produced molecular genetic evidence for the existence of a gene that influences sexual orientation in men (Hamer et al., 1993).

Hamer's group began by extending the family studies described in chapter 12 of this book. They found an increased incidence of homosexuality among the male relatives of gay men, not only among brothers as previously reported, but also among uncles and male cousins. Most interestingly, however, it was only relatives linked through the female line, that is, maternal uncles and the sons of maternal aunts, who had an increased likelihood of being gay.

This "sex-linked" pattern of inheritance suggests the possibility that a gene on the X chromosome might influence sexual orientation in men. The same pattern is seen for some other traits such as anomalous color vision, which is caused by genes on the X chromosome. The reason for the maternal inheritance pattern in such cases is that men always inherit their X chromosome from their mothers. Generally the mother has a gene causing the anomalous trait on one of her two X chromosomes and a gene for the usual condition (for example, regular color vision) on the other. Thus each of her sons stands a 50% chance of inheriting the anomalous gene.

To investigate this possibility further, Hamer and his colleagues examined the DNA from the X chromosomes of a large number of gay men. To sequence (analyze the genetic code of) the entire X chromosome would be an impossibly arduous task. They therefore took advantage of the existence of "markers"—locations on the chromosome where different people are known to have slightly different DNA sequences, which can be recognized by simple biochemical procedures. If two unrelated men are selected, any marker is likely to differ between the two. If two brothers are selected, there is about a 50% chance that any marker will be the same. This is because each brother inherits the marker randomly from one of the two X chromosomes of his mother, and so half of the time they will both inherit the same one. If two gay brothers are selected, then the chances will also be 50%, unless the markers happen to be near the location of a gene influencing sexual orientation. In that case, the chances of the marker being the same in the two brothers will be even higher than 50%, because the two brothers are likely to have both inherited DNA in this region from the same maternal chromosome, namely the chromosome that carried the version of the gene predisposing to homosexuality.

Hamer and his colleagues found that a cluster of markers at one end of the X chromosome, in a region with the technical name of Xq28, was shared by gay brothers at a rate higher than 50%. The statistical analysis showed that this observation was extremely unlikely to have been caused by chance. Rather, it is likely that a gene somewhere in the Xq28 region of the X chromosome predisposes men to be either gay or straight.

The significance of this finding to our understanding of sexual orientation can hardly be overestimated. Although the gene itself has not yet been isolated and sequenced, it probably will be found within a few years. When this happens, it will be possible to ask how and when the gene works. Does it, for example, influence the development of those brain regions—the hypothalamus in particular—that are believed to play a role in generating our sexual feelings and behavior?

The gene in the Xq28 region is probably only one of a number of genes that influence sexual orientation in men, but the discovery will aid the search for the others. Even more important, the identification of the genes will assist the search for the nongenetic factors that undoubtedly play a role in molding our sexual orientation.

Hamer's group—in particular his colleague Angela Pattatucci—are actively searching for genes that influence sexual orientation in women. That such genes exist is indicated by the results of the family and twin studies described in this book. The identification of the genes would be a major advance in the biology of female sexuality. Too often in the past this field has been neglected or hampered by technical problems such as the unavailability of brain tissue from women who were known to have been lesbian. Yet attempting to understand men while ignoring women is like trying to understand day while ignoring night—an impossibility, because each exists only by virtue of the other.

Reference

Hamer, D. H., Hu, S., Magnuson, V. L., Hu, N., and Pattatucci, A. M. L. (1993) A linkage between DNA markers on the X-chromosome and male sexual orientation. *Science* 261:321–337.

Sources and Further Reading

Chapter 2

Dawkins, R. (1989) *The Selfish Gene*. 2nd Edition. Oxford: Oxford University Press.

Hamilton, W. D. (1964) The genetical evolution of social behaviour. *Journal of Theoretical Biology* 7: 1–52.

Hrdy, S. B. (1977) *The Langurs of Abu: Female and Male Strategies of Reproduction*. Cambridge, Massachusetts: Harvard University Press.

Kelley, S. E., Antonovics, J., and Schmitt, J. (1988) A test of the short-term advantage of sexual reproduction. *Nature* 331: 714–717.

Kondrashov, A. S. (1988) Deleterious mutations and the evolution of sexual reproduction. *Nature* 336: 435–440.

Muller, H. J. (1964) The relation of recombination to mutational advance. *Mutation Research* 1: 2–9.

Trivers, R. L. (1985) *Social Evolution*. Menlo Park, California: Benjamin/Cummings.

Chapter 3

Imperato-McGinley, J., Guerrero, L., Gautier, T., and Peterson, R.E. (1974) Steroid 5-alpha-reductase deficiency in man: an inherited form of male pseudo-hermaphroditism. *Science* 186: 1213–1215.

Johnson, M., and Everitt, B. (1988) *Essential Reproduction*. 3rd Edition. Oxford: Blackwell. (An unusually well-written and concise textbook of reproductive physiology, it covers the areas of sexual biology, especially the ovarian cycle, pregnancy and birth, that are not dealt with in this book.)

Koopman, P., Gubbay, J., Vivian, N., Goodfellow, P., and Lovell-Badge, R. (1991) Male development of chromosomally female mice transgenic for Sry. *Nature* 351: 117–121. (Sry is another name for the sex-determining gene TDF.)

Sinclair, A. H., Berta, P., Palmer, M. S., Hawkins, J. R., Griffiths, B. L., Smith, M. J., Foster, J. W., Frischauf, A. M., Lovell-Badge, R., and Goodfellow, P. N.

(1990) A gene from the human sex-determining region encodes a protein with homology to a conserved DNA-binding motif. *Nature* 346: 240–242.

Chapter 4

Olds, J., and Milner, P. (1954) Positive reinforcement produced by electrical stimulation of the septal area and other regions of the rat brain. *Journal of Comparative and Physiological Psychology* 47: 419–427.

Groves, P. M., and Rebec, G. V. (1988) *Introduction to Biological Psychology.* 3rd Edition. Dubuque: Wm. C. Brown. (A highly readable introduction to the study of brain function and behavior.)

Chapter 5

Swanson, L. W. (1987) The hypothalamus. In *Handbook of Chemical Neuroanatomy, Vol. 5,* pp. 1–124 (Björklund, A., Hökfelt, T., and Swanson, L.W., eds.) Amsterdam: Elsevier. (A mine of information about the rat's hypothalamus, though not especially light reading.)

Chapter 6

Breedlove, S. M. (1986) Cellular analysis of hormone influence on motoneuronal development and function. *Journal of Neurobiology* 17: 157–166. (By the ingenious application of genetic techniques, Breedlove provides evidence that the death of motor neurons in the female rat's spinal cord is secondary to the atrophy of the muscles that they innervate.)

Breedlove, S. M., and Arnold, A. P. (1983) Hormonal control of a developing neuromuscular system: I. Complete demasculinization of the male rat spinal nucleus of the bulbocavernosus using the antiandrogen flutamide. II. Sensitive periods for the androgen induced masculinization of the rat spinal nucleus of the bulbocavernosus. *Journal of Neuroscience* 3: 417–423, 424–432.

Darling, C. A., Davidson, J. K., and Conway-Welch, C. (1990) Female ejaculation: perceived origins, the Grafenberg spot/area, and sexual responsiveness. *Archives of Sexual Behavior* 19: 29–47.

Darling, C. A., Davidson, J. K., and Hennings, D. A. (1991) The female sexual response revisited: understanding the multiorgasmic experience in women. *Archives of Sexual Behavior* 20: 527–540.

Murphy, M. R., Checkley, S. A., Seckl, J. R., and Lightman, S. L. (1990) Naloxone inhibits oxytocin release at orgasm in man. *Journal of Clinical Endocrinology and Metabolism* 71: 1056–1058.

Voeller, B. (1991) AIDS and heterosexual anal intercourse. *Archives of Sexual Behavior* 20: 233–276. (Although written from the perspective of HIV transmission, this article includes a valuable survey of the literature on heterosexual anal intercourse.)

Chapter 7

Dixson, A. F., and Lloyd, S. A. C. (1989) Effects of male partners upon proceptivity in ovariectomized estradiol-treated marmosets (*Callithrix jacchus*). *Hormones and Behavior* 23: 211–220. (Analyzes the role of eye contact.)

Goldman, S., and Nottebohm, F. (1983) Neuronal production, migration and differentiation in a vocal control nucleus of the adult female canary brain. *Proceedings of the National Academy of the U.S.A.* 80: 2390–2394.

Gurney, M. (1981) Hormonal control of cell form and number in the zebra finch song system. *Journal of Neuroscience* 1: 658–673.

Pomerantz, S. M., Roy, M. M., and Goy, R. W. (1988) Social and hormonal influences on behavior of adult male, female and pseudohermaphroditic rhesus monkeys. *Hormones and Behavior* 22: 219–230. (Analyzes sexual behavior in monkey "three-ways.")

Chapter 8

Bridges, R.S. (1984) A quantitative analysis of the roles of dosage, sequence, and duration of estradiol and progesterone exposure in the regulation of maternal behavior in the rat. *Endocrinology* 114: 930–940.

Bridges, R. S., DiBiase, R., Loundes, D. D., and Doherty, P. C. (1985) Prolactin stimulation of maternal behavior in female rats. *Science* 227: 782–784.

Ehrhardt, A. A., Meyer-Bahlburg, H. F. L., Rosen, L. R., Feldman, J. F., Veridiano, N. P., Elkin, E. J., and McEwen, B. S. (1989) The development of gender-related behavior in females following prenatal exposure to diethylstilbestrol (DES). *Hormones and Behavior* 23: 526–541.

Gibber, J. R. (1981) *Infant-directed behaviors in male and female rhesus monkeys.* Ph.D. Thesis, University of Wisconsin, Madison, Dept. of Psychology.

Insel, T. R. (1990) Oxytocin and mammalian behavior. In *Mammalian Parenting* (see Krasnegor and Bridges).

Krasnegor, N. A., and Bridges, R. S., eds. (1990) *Mammalian Parenting.* New York: Oxford University Press. (A collection of articles that describe parental, especially maternal behavior in a variety of mammalian species including humans, and analyze the neurobiological and hormonal mechanisms that generate it.)

Modney, B. K., and Hatton, G. I. (1990) Motherhood modifies magnocellular neuronal interrelationships in functionally meaningful ways. In *Mammalian Parenting* (see Krasnegor and Bridges).

Money, J., and Ehrhardt, A. A. (1972) *Man and Woman, Boy and Girl.* Baltimore: Johns Hopkins University Press. (Especially relevant to this chapter is the section on the gender-specific and maternal behavior of girls with congenital adrenal hyperplasia, pp. 98–103. It should be noted that the authors' statement that the syndrome did not cause an increase in homosexuality in adulthood had to be amended when more patients were studied, as detailed in chapter 12 of this book).

Terkel, J., and Rosenblatt, J. S. (1972) Humoral factors underlying maternal behavior at parturition. *Journal of Comparative and Physiological Psychology* 80: 365–371.

Chapter 9

Allen, L. S., Hines, M., Shryne, J. E., and Gorski, R. A. (1989) Two sexually dimorphic cell groups in the human brain. *Journal of Neuroscience* 9: 497–506.

Cherry, J. A., and Baum, M. J. (1990) Effects of lesions of a sexually dimorphic nucleus in the preoptic/anterior hypothalamic area on the expression of androgen- and estrogen-dependent sexual behaviors in male ferrets. *Brain Research* 522: 191–203.

Cohen, R. S., and Pfaff, D. W. (1992) Ventromedial hypothalamic neurons in the mediation of long-lasting effects of estrogen on lordosis behavior. *Progress in Neurobiology* 38: 423–453.

Gorski, R. A., Harlan, R. E., Jacobson, C. D., Shryne, J. E., and Southam, A. M. (1980) Evidence for a morphological sex difference within the medial preoptic area of the rat brain. *Journal of Comparative Neurology* 193: 529–539.

Hennessey, A. C., Wallen, K., and Edwards, D. A. (1986) Preoptic lesions increase display of lordosis by male rats. *Brain Research* 370: 21–28.

Oomura, Y., Aou, S., Koyama, Y., and Yoshimatsu, H. (1988) Central control of sexual behavior. *Brain Research Bulletin* 20: 863–870. (Describes results of electrical stimulation and recording experiments in macaque monkeys.)

Perachio, A. A., Marr, L. D., and Alexander, M. (1979) Sexual behavior in male rhesus monkeys elicited by electrical stimulation of preoptic and hypothalamic areas. *Brain Research* 177: 127–144.

Sachs, B. D., and Meisel, R. L. (1988) The physiology of male sexual behavior. In *The Physiology of Reproduction* (Knobil, E., and Neill, J.D., eds.). New York: Raven Press, pp. 1393–1485.

Slimp, J. C., Hart, B. L., and Goy, R. W. (1978) Heterosexual, autosexual and social behavior of adult male rhesus monkeys with medial preoptic-anterior hypothamic lesions. *Brain Research* 142: 105–122.

Swaab, D. F., and Fliers, E. (1985) A sexually dimorphic nucleus in the human brain. *Science* 228: 1112–1114. (Two subsequent studies failed confirm that the nucleus described by Swaab and Fliers—"SDN-POA," "INAH 1," or "nucleus intermedius"—is in fact sexually dimorphic.)

Thornton, J. E., Nock, B., McEwen, B. S., and Feder, H. H. (1986) Estrogen induction of progestin receptors in microdissected hypothalamic and limbic nuclei of female guinea pigs. *Neuroendocrinology* 43: 182–188.

Chapter 10

Anderson, R. H., Fleming, D. E., Rhees, R. W., and Kinghorn, E. (1986) Relationships between sexual activity, plasma testosterone, and the volume of the sexually dimorphic nucleus of the preoptic area in prenatally stressed and non-stressed rats. *Brain Research* 370: 1–10.

Berenbaum, S. A., and Hines, M. (1992) Early androgens are related to childhood sex-typed toy preferences. *Psychological Science* 3: 203–206.

Döhler, K.-D., Coquelin, A., Davis, F., Hines, M., Shryne, J. E., and Gorski, R. A. (1984) Pre- and postnatal influence of testosterone propionate and diethylstilbestrol on differentiation of the sexually dimorphic nucleus of the preoptic area in male and female rats. *Brain Research* 302: 291–295.

Dodson, R. E., Shryne, J. E., and Gorski, R. A. (1988) Hormonal modification of the number of total and late-arising neurons in the central part of the medial preoptic nucleus of the rat. *Journal of Comparative Neurology* 275: 623–629. (Uses ^{3}H-thymidine autoradiography to examine the influence of androgen levels on the generation and survival of neurons in the sexually dimorphic nucleus.)

Gladue, B. A., and Clemens, L. G. (1978) Androgenic influences on feminine sexual behavior in male and female rats: defeminization blocked by prenatal androgen. *Endocrinology* 103: 1702–1709.

Goy, R. W. (1981) Differentiation of male social traits in female rhesus macaques by prenatal treatment with androgens: variation in type of androgen, duration and timing of treatment. In *Fetal Endocrinology* (Novy, M. J., and Resko, J. A., eds.). New York: Academic Press, pp. 319–339.

Goy, R. W., Wallen, K., and Goldfoot, D. A. (1974) Social factors affecting the development of mounting behavior in male rhesus monkeys. In *Reproductive Behavior* (Montagna, W., and Sadler, W. A., eds.). New York: Plenum Press, pp. 223–247.

Meisel, R. L., and Ward, I. L. (1981) Fetal female rats are masculinized by male littermates located caudally in the uterus. *Science* 213: 239–242.

Moore, C. L. (1984) Maternal contribution to the development of masculine sexual behavior in laboratory rats. *Developmental Psychobiology* 17: 347–356. (Deals with the effects of sex-specific anogenital licking.)

Ward, I. L. (1972) Prenatal stress feminizes and demasculinizes the behavior of males. *Science* 143: 212–218.

Ward, I. L. (1992) Sexual behavior: the product of perinatal hormonal and prepubertal social factors. In *Handbook of Behavioral Neurobiology, Vol. 11.* (Gerall, A. A., Moltz, H., and Ward, I. L., eds.). New York: Plenum Press.

Ward, I. L., and Weisz, J. (1980) Maternal stress alters plasma testosterone in fetal males. *Science* 207: 328–329.

Chapter 11

Allen, L. S., and Gorski, R. A. (1991) Sexual dimorphism of the anterior commissure and massa intermedia of the human brain. *Journal of Comparative Neurology* 312: 97–104

Allen, L. S., Richey, M. F., Chai, Y. M., and Gorski, R. A. (1991) Sex differences in the corpus callosum of the living human being. *Journal of Neuroscience* 11: 933–942.

de Lacoste-Utamsing, M. C., and Holloway, R. L. (1982) Sexual dimorphism in the human corpus callosum. *Science* 216: 1431–1432.

Frank, L. G., Glickman, S. E., and Licht, P. (1991) Fatal sibling aggression, precocial development, and androgens in neonatal spotted hyenas. *Science* 252: 702–704.

Hines, M., Allen, L. S., and Gorski, R. A. (1992) Sex differences in subregions of the medial nucleus of the amygdala and the bed nucleus of the stria terminalis of the rat. *Brain Research* 579: 321–326.

Hines, M., Chiu, L., McAdams, L. A., Bentler, P. M., and Lipcamon, J. (1992) Cognition and the corpus callosum: verbal fluency, visuospatial ability and language lateralization related to midsagittal surface areas of callosal subregions. *Behavioral Neuroscience* 106: 3–14.

Imperato-McGinley, J., Pichardo, M., Gautier, T., Voyer, D., and Bryden, M. P. (1991) Cognitive abilities in androgen-insensitive subjects: comparison with control males and females from the same kindred. *Clinical Endocrinology* 34: 341–347.

Kerns, K. A., and Berenbaum, S. A. (1991) Sex differences in spatial ability in children. *Behavior Genetics* 21: 383–396.

McGregor, A., and Herbert, J. (1992) Differential effects of excitotoxic basolateral and corticomedial lesions of the amygdala on the behavioural and endocrine responses to either sexual or aggression-promoting stimuli in the male rat. *Brain Research* 574: 9–20.

Resnick, S. M., Berenbaum, S. A., Gottesman, I. I., and Bouchard, T. J. (1986) Early hormonal influences on cognitive functioning in congenital adrenal hyperplasia. *Developmental Psychology* 22: 191–198.

Shakespeare, W. (?1591) *Henry the Sixth, Part Three.* London: Penguin Books, 1981. (See Act V, scene vi, for an account of the future King Richard's dental problems.)

Wittig, M. A., and Petersen, A. C., eds. (1979) *Sex-Related Differences in Cognitive Functioning.* New York: Academic Press.

Chapter 12

Historical and General

Freud, S. (1905) *Three Essays on the Theory of Sexuality.* In: *Standard Edition of the Complete Psychological Works of Sigmund Freud, Vol. 7.* London: Hogarth Press, 1953, pp. 125–243.

Isay, R. A. (1989) *Being Homosexual.* New York: Farrar, Straus, Giroux.

Kennedy, H. (1988) *Ulrichs: The Life and Works of Karl Heinrich Ulrichs, Pioneer of the Modern Gay Movement.* Boston: Alyson Publications.

Kinsey, A. C., Pomeroy, W. B., and Martin, C. E. (1948) *Sexual Behavior in the Human Male.* Philadephia: W. B. Saunders.

Kinsey, A. C., Pomeroy, W. B., Martin, C. E., and Gebhard, P. H. (1953) *Sexual Behavior in the Human Female.* Philadelphia: W. B. Saunders.

Genetic Studies

Bailey, J. M., and Pillard, R. C. (1991) A genetic study of male sexual orientation. *Archives of General Psychiatry* 48: 1089–1096.

Bailey, J. M., Pillard, R. C., and Agyei, Y. (1993) A genetic study of female sexual orientation. *Archives of General Psychiatry* (in press).

Eckert, E. D., Bouchard, T. J., Bohlen, J., and Heston, L. L. (1986) Homosexuality in monozygotic twins reared apart. *British Journal of Psychiatry* 148: 421–425.

Pillard, R. C., and Weinrich, J. D. (1986) Evidence of familial nature of male homosexuality. *Archives of General Psychiatry* 43: 808–812.

Schiavi, R. C., Theilgaard, A., Owen, D. R., and White, D. (1988) Sex chromosome anomalies, hormones, and sexuality. *Archives of General Psychiatry* 45: 19–24.

Whitam, F. L., Diamond, M., and Martin, J. (1993) Homosexual orientation in twins: a report on 61 pairs and 3 triplet sets. *Archives of Sexual Behavior* (in press).

Childhood Traits

Bell, A. P., Weinberg, M. S., and Hammersmith, S. K. (1981) *Sexual Preference: Its Development in Men and Women.* New York: Simon and Schuster. (The childhood of lesbians and gay men, based on a large retrospective survey conducted in the San Francisco area in the 1970s.)

Green, R. (1985) Gender identity in childhood and later sexual orientation: follow-up of seventy-eight males. *American Journal of Psychiatry* 142: 339–341.

Green, R. (1987) *The "Sissy-Boy Syndrome" and the Development of Homosexuality.* New Haven: Yale University Press.

Mulaikal, R. M., Migeon, C. J., and Rock, J. A. (1987) Fertility rates in female patients with congenital adrenal hyperplasia due to 21-hydroxylase deficiency. *New England Journal of Medicine* 316: 178–182. (See also the commentary by D. D. Federman, pp. 209–210.)

Money, J., Schwartz, M., and Lewis, V. G. (1984) Adult erotosexual status and fetal hormonal masculinization and demasculinization: 46,XX congenital virilizing adrenal hyperplasia and 46,XY androgen-insensitivity syndrome compared. *Psychoneuroendocrinology* 9: 405–414.

Weinrich, J. D., Grant, I., Jacobson, D. L., Robinson, S. R., and McCutchan, J. A. (1993) On the effects of childhood gender nonconformity on adult genito-erotic role and AIDS exposure. *Archives of Sexual Behavior* (in press).

Whitam, F. L., and Mathy, R. M. (1986) *Male Homosexuality in Four Societies: Brazil, Guatemala, Philippines, and the United States.* New York: Praeger.

Zuger, B. (1984) Early effeminate behavior in boys: outcome and significance for homosexuality. *Journal of Nervous and Mental Disease* 172: 90–97.

Cognitive Studies

Gladue, B. A., Beatty, W. W., Larson, J., and Staton, R. D. (1990) Sexual orientation and spatial ability in men and women. *Psychobiology* 18: 101–108.

Lindesay, J. (1987) Laterality shift in homosexual men. *Neuropsychologia* 25: 965–969.

McCormick, C. M., and Witelson, S. F. (1991) A cognitive profile of homosexual men compared to heterosexual men and women. *Psychoneuroendocrinology* 16: 459–473.

McCormick, C. M., Witelson, S. F., and Kingstone, E. (1990) Left-handedness in homosexual men and women: neuroendocrine implications. *Psychoneuroendocrinology* 15: 69–76.

Sanders, G., and Ross-Field, L. (1986) Sexual orientation and visuo-spatial ability. *Brain and Cognition* 5: 280–290.

Brain Studies

Allen, L. S., and Gorski, R. A. (1992) Sexual orientation and the size of the anterior commissure in the human brain. *Proceedings of the National Academy of Sciences of the U.S.A.* 89: 7199–7202.

Dörner, G., Rohde, W., Stahl, F., Krell, L., and Masius, W. G. (1975) A neuroendocrine predisposition for homosexuality in men. *Archives of Sexual Behavior* 4: 1–8. (This study reports an anomalous luteinizing hormone response to estrogen in homosexual men.)

Hendricks, S. E., Graber, B., and Rodriguez-Sierra, J. F. (1989) Neuroendocrine responses to exogenous estrogen: no differences between heterosexual and homosexual men. *Psychoneuroendocrinology* 14: 177–185. (A failure to confirm Dörner's findings—see above).

LeVay, S. (1991) A difference in hypothalamic structure between heterosexual and homosexual men. *Science* 253: 1034–1037.

Stress Hypothesis

Bailey, J. M., Willerman, L., and Parks, C. (1991) A test of the maternal stress theory of human male homosexuality. *Archives of Sexual Behavior* 20: 277–293. (Contrary to Dörner's hypothesis, this study reports that women who have had a gay and a straight son do not recall different levels of stress during the two pregnancies.)

Dörner, G., Geier, T., Ahrens, L., Krell, L., Münx, G., Sieler, H., Kittner, E., and Müller, H. (1980) Prenatal stress as possible aetiogenetic factor of homosexuality in human males. *Endokrinologie* 75: 365–386. (Reports a greater incidence of homosexuality among men born during the Second World War.)

Dörner, G., Schenk, B., Schmiedel, B., and Ahrens, L. (1983) Stressful events in prenatal life of bi- and homosexual men. *Experimental and Clinical Endocrinology* 81: 83–87.

Ellis, L., Ames, M. A., Peckham, W., and Burke, D. (1988) Sexual orientation of human offspring may be altered by severe maternal stress during pregnancy. *Journal of Sex Research* 25: 152–157. (Offers partial support for the stress hypothesis.)

Homosexuality and Evolution

Hutchinson, G. E. (1959) A speculative consideration of certain possible forms of sexual selection in man. *American Naturalist* 93: 81–91.

Ruse, M. (1981) Are there gay genes? Sociobiology and homosexuality. *Journal of Homosexuality* 6: 5–34.

Weinrich, J. D. (1987) A new sociobiological theory of homosexuality applicable to societies with universal marriage. *Ethology and Sociobiology* 8: 37–47.

Wilson, E. O. (1975) *Sociobiology: The New Synthesis*. Cambridge, Massachusetts: Harvard University Press. (Discusses homosexuality in terms of kin selection theory, p.555.)

Chapter 13

Blanchard, R., (1985) Typology of male-to-female transsexualism. *Archives of Sexual Behavior* 14: 247–261.

Diamond, M. (1982) Sexual identity, monozygotic twins reared in discordant sex roles and a BBC follow-up. *Archives of Sexual Behavior* 11: 181–186. (Provides some follow-up information on the sex-reassigned twin initially described by Money and Ehrhardt.)

Imperato-McGinley, J., Miller, M., Wilson, J. D., Peterson, R. E., Shackleton, C., and Gajdusek, D. C. (1991) A cluster of male pseudohermaphrodites with 5-alpha-reductase deficiency in Papua New Guinea. *Clinical Endocrinology* 34: 293–298.

Imperato-McGinley, J., Peterson, R. E., Gautier, T., and Sterla, E. (1979) Androgens and the evolution of male-gender identity among male pseudohermaphrodites with 5-alpha-reductase deficiency. *New England Journal of Medicine* 300: 1233–1237.

Leavitt, F., and Berger, J. C. (1990) Clinical patterns among male transsexual candidates with erotic interest in males. *Archives of Sexual Behavior* 19: 491–505.

Money, J., and Ehrhardt, A. A. (1972) *Man and Woman, Boy and Girl: The Differentiation and Dimorphism of Gender Identity from Conception to Maturity*. Baltimore: Johns Hopkins University Press.

Tsoi, W. F. (1990) Developmental profile of 200 male and 100 female transsexuals in Singapore. *Archives of Sexual Behavior* 19: 595–605.

Epilogue

Locke, J. (1690) *An Essay Concerning Human Understanding*. Chicago: Henry Regnery Company, 1956.

Sterne, L. (1759–1767) *The Life and Opinions of Tristram Shandy, Gentleman*. Boston, Houghton Mifflin Company, 1965. (Sterne's comic masterpiece applies Locke's philosophy to the construction of a life, with predictably disastrous results.)

Chapter Titles

The chapter titles are taken from, or based on, the following poems or plays of Shakespeare:

Chapter 1. Thou, Nature, Art My Goddess: *King Lear, I,ii*
Chapter 2. Time's Millioned Accidents: *Sonnet 115*
Chapter 3. For a Woman Wert Thou First Created: *Sonnet 20*
Chapter 4. What's in the Brain that Ink May Character?: *Sonnet 108*
Chapter 5. The Womby Vaultage: *Henry the Fifth, II,iv*
Chapter 6. The Beast with Two Backs: *Othello I,i*
Chapter 7. A Joy Proposed: *Sonnet 129*
Chapter 8. The Child-Changed Mother: *King Lear, IV,vii*
Chapter 9. The Generation of Still-Breeding Thoughts: *Richard the Second, V,v*
Chapter 10. My Brain I'll Prove the Female: *Richard the Second, V,v*
Chapter 11. In All Suits Like a Man: *The Taming of the Shrew, Ind.,i*
Chapter 12. So Full of Shapes Is Fancy: *Twelfth Night, I,i*
Chapter 13. Wrapped in a Woman's Hide: *Henry the Sixth, Part Three, I,iv*
Epilogue. Two Artificial Gods: *A Midsummer Night's Dream, III,ii*

Glossary

The meaning of a term given here refers primarily to its use in this book, and is not necessarily a general definition.

ablation Destruction for experimental purposes.

activational effect An effect of a hormone on brain function in adulthood that lasts only as long as the hormone is present (contrast *organizational effect*).

5-alpha-reductase The enzyme responsible for the conversion of testosterone into dihydrotesterone, present in skin and some other tissues.

amino acids The building blocks of peptides and proteins: glutamate, lysine, etc.

amygdala A group of nuclei in the basal forebrain concerned with the processing of sensory inputs for the generation of aggressive, sexual, and other emotion-laden behaviors.

androgens A class of gonadal steroids, including testosterone, whose typical hormonal action is to drive development in a male direction.

antagonist A drug that hinders the action of a natural substance such as a neurotransmitter or hormone by blocking the receptors for that substance.

anterior commissure A bundle of axons connecting the left and right hemispheres of the cerebral cortex, similar in function to the corpus callosum, but much smaller.

anus The exit of the digestive tract; like the penis, it combines excretory and sexual functions.

aromatase An enzyme capable of transforming androgens into estrogens.

asexual reproduction   Reproduction by one individual without any genetic contribution from another individual.

atomy (Shakespeare)   A mite or other diminutive creature.

autoradiography   The visualization of radioactively-labeled compounds in histological sections by the exposure of an overlying photographic emulsion.

autosomes   The chromosomes other than the sex chromosomes.

AVPV   The anteroventral periventricular nucleus: a nucleus at the front of the hypothalamus involved in the regulation of the estrous cycle.

axon   The single long fiber that carries impulses from a neuron's cell body to the axon's terminals, where it forms synapses with other neurons.

bisexuality   Sexual feelings or behavior directed toward both sexes.

castration   Removal of the gonads, especially in males. Psychoanalysts sometimes use the word to mean removal of the penis.

cell-autonomous   Occurring by virtue of instructions intrinsic to each cell.

center   A brain region (often a nucleus) thought of in terms of its distinct role in mental life or behavior.

child-changed (Shakespeare)   Changed by one's child.

chromosome   A rodlike structure within the nuclei of cells that carries a large number of the organism's genes in a fixed sequence.

clitoris   A component of the female external genitalia: a protuberance lying in front of the urethra where the labia minora fuse at the midline. It is an erectile organ and a major site of sexual excitability.

cognitive   Pertaining to the mental basis of knowledge and perception. The word is increasingly being applied to mental processes in general.

coitus or **coition**   Sexual intercourse.

congenital adrenal hyperplasia   A genetic abnormality of steroid biosynthesis that leads to excess secretion of androgens by the adrenal gland during fetal life, and hence to partial masculinization of female fetuses (also known as the adrenogenital syndrome).

Coolidge effect   Shortening of the refractory period for sexual excitability by the introduction of a new partner.

cooperativity A positive interaction between events, such that the more frequently events occur the greater the effect of each event.

copulation Sexual intercourse; the term is generally used for sex in animals rather than humans.

corpus callosum The main axonal pathway interconnecting the left and right hemispheres of the cerebral cortex.

cortex A sheet-like expanse of gray matter on the surface of the brain made up of several layers of neurons.

corticosteroids A group of steroid hormones produced by the adrenal gland that do not play a role in the regulation of sexual behavior or development.

critical period A period of plasticity in the development of some aspect of brain organization, during which it is susceptible to modification by hormonal manipulation, environmental influence, etc.

default The absence of a specific signal or instruction.

dihydrotestosterone An androgen, more potent than testosterone, synthesized from the latter in certain tissues such as the skin.

disruptive selection An evolutionary process in which a population that is more-or-less uniform with respect to a particular attribute splits into two populations that differ from each other in this same attribute.

DNA Deoxyribonucleic acid: the chemical substrate of heredity.

double foot-clasp mount The style of mounting shown by a mature male monkey, in which he raises himself off the ground by grasping his partner's legs with his feet.

ejaculation In men, the forceful expulsion of semen from the penis at orgasm. In some women there is a comparable release of fluid at orgasm, probably from glands homologous to the male prostate.

endorphins Natural brain peptides that have actions similar to the opiate class of drugs.

enzyme A protein that catalyzes (promotes) a specific biochemical reaction.

erection Expansion and hardening by engorgement with blood.

erotic Involving sexual feelings.

estradiol The major estrogenic steroid.

estrogens   A class of gonadal steroids produced by the granulosa cells of the ovarian follicles. Estrogens are responsible for the completion of female sexual development at puberty, and play a key role in the menstrual cycle and pregnancy. In males, estrogens are synthesized from androgens by some brain cells and play a role in the male sexual development of the brain.

estrous cycle   The sexual cycle in female animals, corresponding to the menstrual cycle in women. It is generally shorter than in humans and marked by major changes in sexual receptivity.

female-typical   Seen more commonly in females than males.

film (Shakespeare)   A very slender thread.

firing   Generation of electrical impulses by a neuron.

fitness   Likelihood that an individual's complement of genes will be perpetuated in future generations.

fluorescent   Capable of being excited by light of one wavelength to emit light of another, longer wavelength.

follicle   The developing oocyte with its surrounding granulosa and thecal cells.

gametes   The single-cell, reproductive stages of organisms that mix their genes in sexual reproduction. In higher animals and plants these take two forms, a small male gamete, or sperm, and a large female gamete, or ovum.

gay   Homosexual (used more frequently of men than women).

gender   This word is not used by itself in this book because it has been given such a variety of contradictory meanings by others. See *sex* and *gender identity*.

gender identity   A person's own sense of his or her own maleness or femaleness.

gene   A unit of heredity, consisting of a stretch of DNA that generally encodes a protein ("coding sequence"), several adjoining regulatory sequences, and some apparently functionless interpolated sequences.

gene expression   the activity of a gene, generally meaning the production of the protein for which it codes.

genitalia   Sex organs, usually excluding the gonads. These are grouped into *internal genitalia* (oviducts, uterus, and cervix in females; epididymis, vas deferens, prostate gland, and seminal vesicles in males) and *external genitalia* (vagina, labia minora, labia majora, and clitoris in females; penis and scrotum in males).

germ line   The succession of dividing cells between a zygote and the gametes of the adult organism.

gestation   Pregnancy.

glans   The head of the penis or clitoris.

glial cells   Any of several kinds of non-neuronal cells in the nervous system.

Golgi's method   A method for visualizing entire neurons by precipitating silver chromate within them.

gonad   The organ that produces gametes: the testis (male) or ovary (female). The gonads also produce sex hormones.

gonadal steroids   Steroids produced by the gonads; sex hormones.

granulosa cells   Cells surrounding the developing ovum that are involved in the production of estrogens.

gray matter   The parts of the brain and spinal cord that contain neurons and synapses; it takes the form either of cortex or nuclei.

heterosexuality   Sexual feelings or behavior directed toward individuals of the opposite sex.

heterozygous   Having different versions of a gene on the two members of a pair of chromosomes.

homosexuality   Sexual feelings or behavior directed toward individuals of one's own sex.

homozygous   Having the same versions of a gene on both members of a pair of chromosomes.

hormone   A chemical secreted by specialized endocrine or neuroendocrine cells that is transported (usually via the bloodstream) to other cells or tissues, where it influences their metabolism or development.

^{3}H-thymidine   Thymidine labeled with tritium, an isotope of hydrogen.

hybridization histochemistry   The use of radioactively labeled DNA or RNA to visualize gene expression in histological sections.

hypothalamus   A small region at the base of the brain containing a number of nuclei involved in the regulation of instinctual drives, cardiopulmonary function, endocrine function, metabolism, food and water balance, and temperature regulation.

immunohistochemistry   The use of antibodies to locate a compound such as a neurotransmitter or hormone in histological sections.

INAH 1–4   The four interstitial nuclei of the anterior hypothalamus. INAH 3 is dimorphic with sex and sexual orientation; INAH 2 may be dimorphic with sex; INAH 1 (also known as the nucleus intermedius) and INAH 4 are probably not dimorphic with either sex or sexual orientation.

intersexual   Anatomically intermediate or ambiguous in sex.

intromission   The insertion of the penis into an orifice such as the vagina.

investment   The expenditure of energy or resources by an organism when that expenditure has some chance of resulting in a later benefit to the organism's reproductive success.

isotope   (as used in this book) A radioactive version of an atom.

joiner   A maker of small wooden articles.

Kallmann's syndrome   A congenital condition characterized by delayed puberty and the absence of the sense of smell.

kin selection   The theory whereby animals may increase their fitness, in the evolutionary sense, by promoting the reproductive success of their relatives.

Klinefelter's syndrome   A syndrome in men caused by the possession of an extra X chromosome. The affected men tend to be tall, of lower-than-average intelligence, and infertile.

labia majora   The tissue folds surrounding the labia minora.

labia minora   The inner tissue folds surrounding the vagina and urethra.

lesbian   Homosexual (of women).

lesion   A region of damage to the brain, occurring by a disease process such as a stroke in humans, or made deliberately in experimental animals with a view to understanding the function of that region.

Leydig cells   Androgen-producing cells of the testis.

lordosis   In rodents and some other animals, a reflex curving of the back into a U-shape that exposes the genitalia and permits intromission.

luteinizing hormone (LH)   A peptide hormone secreted by the pituitary gland that induces the final maturation of the developing oocyte. In males it stimulates testosterone production by the Leydig cells of the testis.

luteinizing hormone–releasing hormone (LHRH)   A peptide hormone synthesized by a specialized set of hypothalamic neurons that is transported by blood vessels to the pituitary gland, where it regulates the secretion of luteinizing hormone.

male-typical   Seen more commonly in males than females.

maternal stress effect   Reduction of male-typical sexual behavior in male rats whose mothers were stressed during pregnancy.

medial   Toward the midline.

medial preoptic area   The portion of the preoptic area closest to the midline.

median   Straddling the midline.

menstrual cycle   The cycle (monthly in humans) in which the uterus alternates between a state suitable for the transport of sperm and a state suitable for the implantation of the embryo.

microelectrode   A metal wire or glass capillary that tapers to an extremely fine tip, used to record the electrical activity of single neurons.

millioned (Shakespeare)   Innumerable.

mitosis   The usual kind of cell division, in which the daughter cells have the same chromosomal makeup as the parent cell.

mosaic   An individual composed of a patchwork of tissues of two or more different genetic origins.

mRNA   Messenger RNA: the form of RNA that acts as a template for the synthesis of proteins.

müllerian duct   The embryonic precursor of the female internal genitalia.

müllerian inhibition hormone (MIH)   A hormone produced by the male gonad during early development that prevents the müllerian duct from developing into the female genital tract.

Muller's ratchet   The stepwise, irreversible increase in the minimum number of harmful mutations in a finite, asexually reproducing population.

mutation   A change in a gene.

naloxone   A synthetic antagonist of opiates and endorphins.

neuroendocrine cells   Cells that combine the functions of neurons and glandular cells.

neuron   A nerve cell.

neurotransmitter   A chemical used for transmission of signals across synapses.

nucleus (plural **nuclei**)   (1) The central compartment of a cell, which contains most of its genetic material. (2) In neuroanatomy, a coherent assembly of neurons recognizable as a discrete structure in the brain. The neurons in a nucleus are generally similar to each other in structure, chemistry, connections, and function.

nucleus intermedius   A nucleus in the human hypothalamus, also known as INAH 1. One group of researchers reported that it is larger in men than women, but two other studies have failed to confirm this.

optic chiasm   The crossing of the two optic nerves: a landmark at the front of the hypothalamus.

organizational effect   A feature of brain organization that is brought about by hormonal means during early development, and which permanently influences an individual's behavior.

orgasm   Sexual climax in either sex: a brief period of intense pleasure and release, with accompanying increase in heart and respiratory rates, sometimes with skin flushes, muscle spasms, or involuntary cries. Accompanied by ejaculation in men and in some women.

ovary   The female gonad, a paired organ within the pelvic cavity that produces ova and sex hormones.

ovulation   The release of the unfertilized ovum from the ovary.

ovum (plural **ova**)   An egg, before or after fertilization. Before fertilization it is a female gamete or *oocyte;* after fertilization it is a zygote.

oxytocin   A peptide hormone synthesized by hypothalamic neurosecretory neurons that plays a role in orgasm, parturition, lactation, and maternal behavior.

paraventricular nucleus   One of the two hypothalamic nuclei that contain oxytocin- and vasopressin-producing neurons (the other is the supraoptic nucleus).

penile   Of the penis.

penis The major component of the male external genitalia, consisting of glans (head) and shaft. The penis contains erectile tissue and is traversed by the urethra. It serves for the voiding of urine, sexual arousal, intromission, and ejaculation of semen. It is derived from the same tissue as the clitoris and labia minora in females.

perianal Around the anus.

peroxidase An enzyme, commonly extracted from horseradish, that is used as a tracer in the brain.

PET Positron emission tomography: a method for functional imaging of the brain.

pituitary gland A gland connected by a stalk to the undersurface of the hypothalamus. It secretes a large number of hormones that regulate the function of other glandular organs, including the gonads and mammary glands.

placental lactogens Prolactin-like hormones produced by the placenta.

preoptic area The frontmost portion of the hypothalamus, from the optic chiasm forward (some authors consider it a separate brain region from the hypothalamus proper).

presenting Female-typical sexual behavior in monkeys: the display of the genital area as a stimulus to mounting. Can be either proceptive (spontaneous) or receptive (evoked by partner's behavior).

proceptive behavior Female-typical behavior that actively solicits sex, for example staring or spontaneous presenting in monkeys, ear-wiggling in rats (contrast with *receptive behavior.*)

progesterone Principal member of a class of steroid hormones (progestins) produced by the ovary that play a role in the menstrual cycle and the maintenance of pregnancy.

prolactin A protein hormone secreted by the pituitary gland that plays a role in milk production and maternal behavior.

psychoanalysis Freud's technique for treating neuroses by bringing to consciousness their supposed origin in the intra- and interpersonal conflicts of early life.

puberty The transition from childhood to sexual maturity.

receptive behavior Female-typical sexual behavior (e.g., lordosis in rats) that is shown in response to the partner's behavior (e.g., mounting) and which permits copulation (contrast with *proceptive behavior*).

receptor   A large molecule, consisting mainly of protein, whose chemical structure allows it to recognize and bind a particular hormone, neurotransmitter, or other small molecule.

refractory period   A period after a physiological response during which that response cannot be elicited.

scrotum   Component of male external genitalia: the sac that encloses the testes. It derives from the same tissue as the labia majora in females.

semen   The fluid ejaculated from the penis at orgasm; it contains sperm along with the secretions of the prostate and other glands.

seminal emission   The discharge of semen into the urethra; usually followed immediately by ejaculation.

Seven Minutes in Heaven   A children's game in which a boy and girl are put in a closet and given this much time to play at making out.

sex   An individual's maleness or femaleness, based primarily on the anatomy of his or her external genitalia.

sex-atypical   More common in the opposite sex.

sex chromosomes   The pair of chromosomes (X and Y) responsible for sex determination.

sex-linked   Inherited along with sex, i.e. by means of genes located on the sex chromosomes.

sexual dimorphism   An anatomical difference between the sexes.

sexually dimorphic nucleus   A nucleus in the medial preoptic area of the rat's hypothalamus that is larger in males than in females.

sexual orientation   The direction of sexual feelings or behavior toward the same sex, the opposite sex, or some combination of the two.

sexual reproduction   A form of reproduction involving the merging of genetic material from two individuals.

sibling   Brother or sister.

sickle-cell anemia   An inherited blood disorder caused by a mutation in the hemoglobin gene.

singleton   Single-born child (not a twin).

sodomy   Has been used variously to describe anal intercourse (whether homosexual or heterosexual), homosexual behavior in general, or any sexual behavior prohibited by a particular jurisdiction.

sociobiology The study of behavior, especially social behavior, from the point of view of the evolutionary mechanisms that generate it.

sperm (or **spermatozoa**) The male gametes: the cellular constituents of semen.

spinner (Shakespeare) A spider.

splenium The enlarged back end of the corpus callosum.

steroids A class of molecules synthesized from cholesterol and consisting of four connected carbon rings.

still-breeding (Shakespeare) Ever-breeding.

straight Heterosexual.

suprachiasmatic nucleus A nucleus of the hypothalamus that regulates the daily cycles of activity, temperature, etc.

supraoptic nucleus One of the two hypothalamic nuclei that contain oxytocin- and vasopressin-producing neurons (the other is the paraventricular nucleus).

sympathetic nervous system A set of motor nerves that originate in ganglia near the spinal cord and innervate involuntary muscles, blood vessels, glands, etc. They use an adrenalin-like compound as a neurotransmitter.

synapse A point of contact between two neurons where the activity of one neuron excites or inhibits the activity of the other.

testis (plural **testes**) or **testicle** The male gonad, a paired organ lying within the scrotum that produces sperm and sex hormones.

testis-determining factor (TDF) The sex-determining gene in mammals. It is located on the Y chromosome and confers maleness by causing the gonads to develop as testes.

testosterone The principal androgenic steroid hormone, synthesized by Leydig cells in the testis and thecal cells in the ovary (in the ovary it is subsequently converted to estrogens).

thalamus A large group of nuclei deep within the cerebral hemispheres. The thalamus controls the inputs to the cerebral cortex and modulates the activity level of the cortex.

thecal cells The outer cells of the ovarian follicle. They synthesize androgens that are subsequently converted into estrogens by the granulosa cells.

third ventricle A slit-shaped ventricle in the midline of the brain that divides the thalamus and hypothalamus into left and right halves.

thymidine A chemical precursor of one of the building blocks of DNA.

trace A strap attached to an animal's collar for drawing a cart.

tracer A compound that is injected into a brain region, taken up by neurons and transported along axons. It is used to delineate neuronal pathways in the brain.

tract An axonal pathway.

transsexuality Discordance between sex and gender identity.

Turner's syndrome A congenital abnormality in women, involving mal-development of the ovaries, caused by the possession of only a single X chromosomes.

urethra The tube through which urine is conveyed from the bladder to the exterior of the body. In males, the ejaculation of semen also takes place through the urethra.

uterine contiguity effect The partial masculinization of female rat festuses by exposure to testosterone secreted by nearby male fetuses.

uterus The womb: site of implantation and development of the embryo.

vagina the sheath-like component of the female external genitalia that forms a passage between the uterus and the exterior. It serves for sexual arousal, penile intromission, passage of sperm and menstrual fluid, and as the last portion of the birth canal.

vasopressin A peptide hormone synthesized by some neurons in the supraoptic and paraventricular nuclei of the hypothalamus that stimulates contraction of blood vessels and the production of concentrated urine by the kidneys.

vasotocin A peptide hormone in submammalian species that is believed to be ancestral to oxytocin and vasopressin.

vaultage Cavern.

ventricle A cavity within the brain filled with cerebrospinal fluid.

ventromedial nucleus A hypothalamic nucleus involved in the generation of female-typical sexual behavior, as well as other functions including the regulation of appetite.

white matter The portions of the brain and spinal cord that contain only axons, not cell bodies or synapses.

wolffian duct   The embryonic precursor of the male internal genitalia.

womby (Shakespeare)   Womb-like.

worm (Shakespeare)   A tick or mite, thought to infect the hands of idle persons.

zygote   The fertilized ovum: the single cell, formed by fusion of male and female gametes, that divides repeatedly to form an embryo.

Index